PHARMACOECONOMICS

Commissioning Editor: Timothy Horne
Project Development Manager: Hannah Kenner
Project Manager: Nancy Arnott
Designer: Erik Bigland
Illustrator: John Marshall

PHARMACOECONOMICS

Edited by

Tom Walley MD FRCP, FRCPI, MRCGP
Professor of Clinical Pharmacology
Prescribing Research Group
Department of Pharmacology and Therapeutics
University of Liverpool, UK

Alan Haycox BA, MA, PhD
Senior Lecturer in health Economics
Prescribing Research Group
Department of Pharmacology and Therapeutics
University of Liverpool, UK

Angela Boland BA, MSc
Research Fellow in Health Economics
Prescribing Research Group
Department of Pharmacology and Therapeutics
University of Liverpool, UK

Foreword by
Professor Alasdair M Breckenridge CBE, MD, FRCP, FRSE
Chairman of Medicine and Healthcare Products Regulatory Agency;
Emeritus Professor of Clinical Pharmacology
University of Liverpool, UK

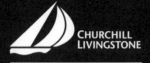
CHURCHILL
LIVINGSTONE

EDINBURGH LONDON NEW YORK OXFORD PHILADELPHIA ST LOUIS SYDNEY
TORONTO 2004

CHURCHILL LIVINGSTONE

© 2004, Elsevier Science Limited. All rights reserved.

The right of Tom Walley, Alan Haycox and Angela Boland be identified as editors of this work has been asserted by them in accordance with the Copyright, Designs and Patents Act 1988

First published 2004

ISBN 0443 07240 X

British Library Cataloguing in Publication Data
A catalogue record for this book is available from the British Library

Library of Congress Cataloging in Publication Data
A catalog record for this book is available from the Library of Congress

Notice
Medical knowledge is constantly changing. Standard safety precautions must be followed, but as new research and clinical experience broaden our knowledge, changes in treatment and drug therapy may become necessary or appropriate. Readers are advised to check the most current product information provided by the manufacturer of each drug to be administered to verify the recommended dose, the method and duration of administration, and contraindications. It is the responsibility of the practitioner, relying on experience and knowledge of the patient, to determine dosages and the best treatment for each individual patient. Neither the Publisher nor the authors assumes any liability for any injury and/or damage to persons or property arising from this publication.

 your source for books, journals and multimedia in the health sciences
www.elsevierhealth.com

The publisher's policy is to use paper manufactured from sustainable forests

Printed in Spain

CONTENTS

Contents

LIST OF CONTRIBUTORS

Pippa Anderson BSc, MSc
Director
Fourth Hurdle Consulting Ltd, London, UK

Adrian Bagust BSc, MIMA, Cmath
Honorary Senior Research Fellow
Prescribing Research Group, Department of Pharmacology and Therapeutics,
University of Liverpool, UK

Angela Boland BA, MSc
Research Fellow in Health Economics
Prescribing Research Group, Department of Pharmacology and Therapeutics,
University of Liverpool, UK

Julia Bottomley PhD
Managing Director
Amygdala Ltd, Letchworth Garden City, UK

Steve Chapman PhD
Professor of Prescribing Studies
Department of Medicines Management, University of Keele, UK

David M. Grant BSc, MBA
Director
Fourth Hurdle Consulting Ltd, London, UK

Alan Haycox BA, MA, PhD
Senior Lecturer in Health Economics
Prescribing Research Group, Department of Pharmacology and Therapeutics,
University of Liverpool, UK

Dyfrig Hughes BPharm, MSc, PhD, MRPharmS
Lecturer in Pharmacoeconomics
Prescribing Research Group, Department of Pharmacology and Therapeutics,
University of Liverpool, UK

Adam Lloyd MPhil
Director
Fourth Hurdle Consulting Ltd, London, UK

Ruth McDonald BA, MSc, CPFA, PhD
NHS/PPP Research Fellow
Department of Applied Social Science, University of Manchester, UK

Antonieta Medina Lara BSc, MSc
Research Fellow in Health Economics
Prescribing Research Group, Department of Pharmacology and Therapeutics,
University of Liverpool, UK

Ruben E Mujica Mota MSc
Research Fellow
Prescribing Research Group, Department of Pharmacology and Therapeutics,
University of Liverpool, UK

Prescribing Research Group,
Department of Pharmacology and Therapeutics, University of Liverpool,
Liverpool L69 3GF
prgroup@liv.ac.uk

Judith Strobl MPH, BSc
Research Fellow
Prescribing Research Group, Department of Pharmacology and Therapeutics,
University of Liverpool, UK

Tom Walley MD FRCP, FRCPI, MRCGP
Professor of Clinical Pharmacology
Prescribing Research Group, Department of Pharmacology and Therapeutics,
University of Liverpool, UK

List of contributors

FOREWORD

The traditional role of health professionals within the healthcare system is changing, and the discipline of pharmacology is at the forefront of these changes. Rapid growth in the drugs bill combined with ever-increasing pressure to control healthcare expenditure inevitably places pharmacoeconomics at the leading edge of thinking with regard to optimal drug use. But what is pharmacoeconomics? Where did this new discipline spring from and what (if anything) is its parentage? What is certain is that issues of cost effectiveness are increasingly being placed alongside issues of clinical effectiveness in determining the desirability of introducing new drugs into the clinician's therapeutic armoury. New developments such as the National Institute for Clinical Excellence emphasise the value placed on clinical and cost assessments at the national level. As health professionals, we need to understand the implications of such developments and to ensure that such analyses are informed by the highest quality clinical evidence available. This requires a closer and more focused collaboration between health professionals and health economists to facilitate the cost-effective use of new drugs. Such a collaborative environment will enable health professionals and health economists to achieve the common aim of efficient and effective delivery of healthcare to patients.

As part of the journey towards achieving this aim, health economists need to 'demystify' their discipline, and this book represents a significant contribution to this objective. The unifying force underlying this book is that health professionals need to understand pharmacoeconomics and health economists need to understand the context in which health professionals operate. The book provides a useful non-technical introduction to pharmacoeconomics and identifies the implications for pharmacoeconomic analyses of the policy context in which the health service operates. It also looks at ways in which economic analyses are being applied to improve resource allocation within health service programmes.

The book also examines how pharmacoeconomic analyses can be incorporated sensitively into the clinical trial. Health professionals will increasingly come across such analyses in their professional literature. This book provides guidance on how to distinguish 'good' analyses from 'bad' ones, and hence how such analyses should be incorporated into health professional decision making.

Each of the contributors to this book is to be congratulated for providing a clear and lucid overview of this complex area of analysis. This book constitutes a significant contribution to this important area of debate.

Professor Alasdair M Breckenridge
Chairman of the Medicines and
Healthcare Products Regulatory Agency and
Emeritus Professor of Clinical Pharmacology,
University of Liverpool, UK
2004

PREFACE

Whether you work as a health professional or as an employee of a pharmaceutical company, you will be aware of the pressures to contain costs in healthcare and how heavily these efforts fall on prescribing. You may feel that health economics equates with cutting costs and services or with trying to justify the high price of a new drug. In either event, you may feel inclined to reject it out of hand. But neither view is correct – health economics and in particular its application to medicines, pharmacoeconomics, has a lot to offer whatever your background and current position. We realised that there were no books that addressed these issues from a European perspective and hence this volume came about.

This book is aimed at the intelligent non-specialist reader who wants some of this subject demystified. We had several aims: to explain basic health economics, to outline the complexities of the health services within which health economics operates and the context of medicine use; to explain the basics of the methods of economic evaluation in relation to medicines; and lastly, to help the reader to understand and evaluate the pharmacoeconomic studies which are becoming increasingly common. We have tried to do this in as jargon-free a manner as possible: whether we have succeeded is for the reader to judge.

Our starting point is to discuss the kind of health services found in Europe, Australia or New Zealand – largely publicly funded through central taxation or social insurance, and with a strong sense of social solidarity. Some of what we say will therefore be less applicable to a reader with a solely North American vision or to someone whose interests lie primarily in developing countries. We have spent more time talking about the nature of these health services than most books dealing with these subjects because we think that the context in which pharmacoeconomics operates is extremely important. We have also centered on the UK NHS partly because of our own backgrounds and because, in terms of how pharmacoeconomics is applied, the UK is one of the more advanced countries. We expect that the reader will not want to read separate books on structures of health services or basic health economics so we have condensed the key points here.

We have tried to explain why pharmacoeconomics has grown in importance in these health services and what roles it may play in the pharmaceutical industry or health service. In this, different authors have stressed their own point of view or perspective (some academic, some industry, some public health service). We do not make any judgments on whether one is more valid than any other; each has its place. We hope that pharmacoeconomics can help bridge the gaps between these perspectives, but to do this it needs to become more scientifically rigorous and to be better understood by target audiences who will not accept flawed studies. We hope readers find this book a useful contribution to this.

Liverpool   TW
2004   AH
                                                                                                    AB

Basics of economics, health economics and pharmacoeconomics

INTRODUCTION

Health services throughout the world are increasingly faced with new demands for healthcare. However, as this demand grows so too do the resource constraints faced by decision makers. By accepting the need for choice and informing that choice by examining the costs and benefits of different drugs, healthcare decision makers find themselves working within the field of **health economics**:

- Health economics analyses the supply and demand for healthcare and provides a structure for understanding the choices made therein.
- **Pharmacoeconomics** adopts and applies the principles and methodologies of health economics to the field of pharmaceutical policy (supply and demand for medicines).

The aim of this book is to ensure that decision makers understand, as far as possible, this area of analysis.

Before we can really understand how the tools of health economics and pharmacoeconomics are used to inform healthcare decision making, it is necessary to first of all introduce their parent discipline, economics.

ECONOMICS

Economics is the science of scarcity and choice. Economists analyse the way in which individuals structure and prioritise their personal consumption in their attempt to maximise welfare within constrained resources. Economics is a skill that we all use on a daily basis in our everyday lives. We use it in the small decisions (do I buy the cheaper chocolate bar or pay a bit more for the nicer one?) and the larger decisions (do I buy the Ferrari or the Lada?). The greater the resource implications arising from the decision, the more detailed our economic scrutiny (we are more careful to balance the 'costs' and 'benefits' when we buy a car than when we buy a chocolate bar). We are also constrained by the resources available to us (our heart says 'Ferrari', our bank manager says 'Lada'). Equally, the comparative benefits derived from the cars will depend on our individual circumstances (the younger driver is more likely to

Concept box 1.1 – Scarcity, choice and prioritisation

Scarcity of resources requires individuals to choose which goods and services they consume. The basis for their choice is the relative value that they place on each good or service. The structure of these relative values is the basis for their system of prioritisation.

Concept box 1.2 – Utility

Utility is the value placed on a good or service by any individual as a measure of its usefulness. Total utility is the value placed on consumption of all goods and services.

value speed whereas the older driver is more likely to value safety). Once we have calculated and compared the costs and benefits of the alternatives available, we then make our decision. If we apply such economic principles in our private lives, then we should also apply them in our professional lives.

Economics might be the discipline behind making choices but why do we have to make choices in the first place? Why can't we have everything we want? The answer is that resources (money, time, people) are scarce and so we want to make the best use of them. If we have unlimited demands but limited resources, we have to make choices. When we try to choose which demands should be satisfied from our scarce resources, we have to set priorities. This is true of organisations as well as individuals, and might be especially true in healthcare systems.

The theoretical basis of classical economics

Classical economics focused on the 'usefulness' that individuals placed on goods and services. This 'usefulness' has come to be known as **'utility'**. Classical economists believed that the:

- utility of individuals was entirely dependent on their personal consumption of goods and services
- welfare of society was merely the sum of the utilities of all the individual members of that society.

The important idea to note here is that this limited definition of personal welfare is entirely related to personal consumption.

This definition has, however, been superseded by a concept of social welfare, which involves the well-being of groups or society as a whole – a collective benefit in welfare economics. The major problem with the concept of social welfare is the lack of any simple measure to evaluate the welfare of different groups of individuals. In classical welfare economics, the test of any

Concept box 1.3 – Compensation and the Pareto principle

The concept of 'compensation' was introduced in response to the Pareto principle (see below). Using this concept, individuals whose utility is diminished could be reimbursed by an amount of money that was sufficient to compensate exactly for any adverse effects (e.g. the increased noise and traffic confusion associated with a new hospital). In this manner, 'losers' from any change can, theoretically, be maintained at their previous levels of utility, as required by the Pareto principle.

The Pareto principle

The vast majority of public projects are likely to make at least some members of the population worse off. Even the development of a new hospital would be unlikely to be welcomed by neighbours, given the increased noise and inconvenience. As such, the Pareto principle – which states that it is impossible to compare the welfare of different individuals and that hence only projects by which everybody gains can be given unambiguous support – was in danger of undermining the practical applicability of welfare economics. For this reason, the concept of 'compensation' was developed.

policy was that it should make at least one person better off and nobody worse off. But few policies in the health and welfare field will not make at least one individual worse off, and so the practical applicability of classical welfare economics was limited.

To overcome this problem, the idea of compensation was introduced, that is, if the gainers from a policy could compensate the losers and still be better off, then the policy could be interpreted unambiguously as leading to an increase in social welfare. It seemed possible to measure welfare losses and gains from the perspective of society as a whole by placing monetary values on individual welfare. This was the beginnings of modern-day cost benefit analysis and is central to the development of health economics and pharmacoeconomics.

HEALTH ECONOMICS

Health economics is basically economics applied to healthcare and it is most commonly used to help decision makers make difficult choices. Health economics:

- analyses the supply and demand for healthcare
- provides a structure for understanding decisions and their consequences.

As decision makers become more familiar with the ideas behind health economics, health providers internationally are routinely using the economic language of the marketplace. They talk of purchasing and providing, buying

Concept box 1.4 – Resources

When we consider the resources available to us, we normally think about financial resources (money in our bank accounts). The economists' definition, however, is far wider and encompasses the time, energy and skills exhibited by the individual together with the buildings and equipment that individual might possess. In this manner, a resource might be consumed (time and effort expended in developing an idea) even if there is no associated financial payment.

and selling, demand and need, costs and benefits, inputs and outputs, and efficiency and **effectiveness**. Such language reflects the new emphasis that is being placed on obtaining the maximum value for money in healthcare. Increasingly, healthcare providers are becoming accountable for showing the value for money obtained from their use of scarce resources.

Healthcare is very different from other goods and services and, unlike most economic markets, the market for healthcare has some unusual characteristics.

Efficiency

The concept of efficiency is central to economic theory. Efficiency measures how well resources are used in order to achieve a desired output. It has a number of different definitions.

Within the field of healthcare, *allocative efficiency* is achieved when we allocate resources to those groups or individuals who can benefit most and no reallocation of resources can generate a greater level of health outcome. For example, allocative efficiency is achieved when statins are given to high-risk patients before patients who are low risk. If there were some high-risk patients who did not receive the drug then allocative efficiency is not achieved because a reallocation of drugs from low- to high-risk patients would mean that a greater level of health outcome could be possible.

Technical efficiency is achieved when the minimum amounts of a resource are used to achieve the desired effect (e.g. 'What is the least expensive way to heal a peptic ulcer?') or when resources are fixed and the greatest benefit is achieved (e.g. 'This year we've used our fixed drugs budget to reduce cardiac deaths by 5% more than we did last year'). In such circumstances, excessive prescribing, such as the provision of unnecessarily long courses of drugs, would lead to technical inefficiency.

In a perfectly functioning market, efficiency is ensured because inefficient providers are forced out of business. This frees up the scarce resources that these inefficient providers used for use by more efficient producers. Health economics takes its theoretical toolkit directly from classical welfare economics, which assumes that the greater the level of competition, the more single-minded the pursuit of profit and hence the greater the level of efficiency.

Concept box 1.5 – Perfect competition

This is a hypothetical situation in which all market power is held in the hands of the consumer because there are so many producers that none of them has power in the marketplace. A producer must operate with maximum efficiency or go out of business as consumers switch their purchasing towards other producers operating at lower cost and hence exhibiting a lower price.

However, within the health service, pure efficiency-seeking behaviour might not be the most important objective. We might, for instance, prioritise caring for dying patients or treating patients with serious disease who have relatively little hope of surviving. We might do this even though we know there are other, more efficient, uses of resources. The role of the health economist might not therefore be to determine where key health services are provided but to provide information that will inform any decision made. However, there are times when we *do* want to know how to use our scarce resources efficiently and to do this we need to analyse the costs and benefits of competing options to identify how to maximise benefits to patients.

It is important to distinguish between efficiency and **affordability**. The amount of resources devoted to any health service is entirely constrained by the willingness of the population served to fund the service. As such, it is important to recognise that health services, both individually and collectively, might be highly efficient but too expensive to support. In large part, the extent to which affordability can outstrip cost effectiveness results largely from the very success of healthcare systems in improving health. Improved levels of health within populations inevitably leads to an increase in average life expectancy, which implies that there are more elderly patients imposing greater demands on the health services. Unfortunately, this enhanced demand is being juxtaposed with a proportionate decrease in the working population, resulting in a dwindling tax base from which to pay for health services (Fig. 1.1). In such circumstances, it is perhaps not surprising that **cost containment** has become a major concern within every healthcare system. Issues underlying the use of **rationing** to constrain the demands placed on healthcare provision are discussed in greater detail in Chapter 3.

Lack of competition and resource constraints within health services

As mentioned above, in a perfectly functioning market the structure of resource allocation is determined through competition between purchasers and providers of both goods and services. In the health service, however, one factor that can lessen competitive forces is the fact that hospitals might be sole suppliers of certain treatments (monopolists) whereas local health authorities or insurers might be sole customers for certain treatments (monopsonists).

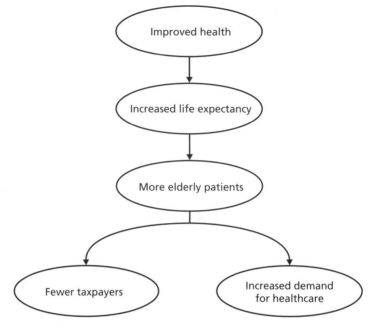

Fig 1.1 How affordability can outstrip cost effectiveness

Concept box 1.6 – Monopolists and monopsonists

A **monopolist** is at the opposite extreme from perfect competition because all market power is in the hands of a single producer. This producer can control the market price and consumers simply have to accept the price as set.

A **monopsonist** is a sole purchaser of goods and services in the marketplace.

When a monopolist (single seller) confronts a monopsonist (single buyer) the resultant price and quantity of goods and services purchased is indeterminate and relates largely to the negotiating power on each side of the marketplace.

Most health services were at least partly founded on the belief that once the existing stock of ill health caused by poor access to healthcare was eliminated, then lower levels of healthcare provision would be required, which would be affordable at a sustainable cost. Unfortunately, experience has shown us that the level of demand, especially in a healthcare system that is free at the point of delivery, will rapidly exceed any nation's ability to fund health services unless some form of restrictions are imposed.

Resource constraints therefore do not necessarily arise from waste in the system. In fact, health services have become far more effective in confronting a far wider range of diseases than in the past. Part of the expansion in the cost of healthcare provision will therefore reflect the valuable extension of healthcare to people who previously were not treatable, together with the provision of higher quality healthcare.

Price signals

The role of price signals and the way in which individuals react to price changes is very important in understanding the market for healthcare. Usually, as the price of a good or service rises, the demand for that good or service by individuals or groups falls. Then, as the price increases, new competitors come into the market because they are attracted by the high price (Fig. 1.2). A natural consequence of this is that competition increases and the price of the good or service inevitably falls. One of the fundamental differences between health and other areas of economics is that some consumers (e.g. patients or doctors) exhibit a reduced sensitivity to price signals and their consumption of healthcare remains reasonably constant even if the price increases. This is mainly because in many health services the costs of healthcare are borne by government or through health insurance schemes. Price signals in the marketplace then become dampened as the price paid by the consumer and the price received by the producer become distorted at the point of service delivery and receipt.

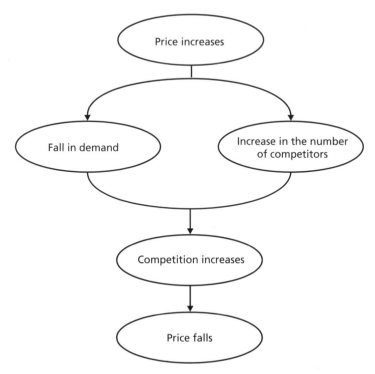

Fig 1.2 The role of price signals

Concept box 1.7 – Definition of need

'Need' has different interpretations. For example, consider a young man who feels that he 'needs' access to Viagra™. This is a 'felt need' and he might express it to his doctor, at which point it becomes an 'expressed need'. The doctor might disagree on the basis that the young man is not likely to benefit greatly and that the drug would be of greater value to other patients ('comparative need'). In addition, the young man might be outside the target group for Viagra™ as established by an independent expert group of health professionals ('normative need').

Definition of need

Classic economics assumes that the individual is the best judge of his or her own welfare. In the field of healthcare, this means that suppliers (e.g. doctors) should provide healthcare in line with consumer (e.g. patient) demand. However, as patients are not usually aware of the best specialist healthcare treatments available, the validity of this assumption must be questioned.

When it comes to healthcare, it is normally accepted in a publicly funded service that the allocation of resources is more appropriately based on patient 'need' rather than patient 'demand'. The problem with having a service based around patient needs is the difficulty that is encountered in defining and measuring the needs of patients for healthcare. Indeed, the very definition of need has been the subject of a broad spectrum of research. It is perhaps sensible to link a patient's need to that individual's ability to benefit from healthcare provision. Unfortunately, identifying a patient's ability to benefit from healthcare provision is likely to be as difficult as defining a patient's need for healthcare. Assessing the health needs of a population through a health needs assessment is an important first step in the prioritisation of health services within local structures.

Definition of health

Defining and measuring health is even more difficult than doing the same for utility or welfare. However, even if we redefine our objective from utility maximisation to health maximisation, we still need a practical measure of health gain so that we can evaluate the comparative values of different ways to treat patients. There might be some simple physical or natural measures we can use (e.g. lives saved or hospital admissions avoided) but sometimes we have to ask individuals (patients, general public, healthcare experts) what they think about various states of health. For instance, is it better to live for 10 years with only one leg or to keep both and only live for 7 years? We can then, using a range of techniques, place values on various states of health and aggregate responses to derive a valuation that is representative of the views

Concept box 1.8 – Definition of health

'Health' has no generally accepted definition and a wide range of physical, mental and social characteristics. The breadth of such characteristics and their essentially subjective nature emphasises the difficulties inherent in deriving an operational definition for this concept.

of society as a whole. Unfortunately, calculating the health gain associated with all treatments in all patient subgroups represents an enormous task, given the wide disparity in patients and healthcare interventions and the rapid dissemination of new treatments and new diseases. We might also get different views depending on who we ask – patients are often more accepting of the limitations of their disease than the general public. Many of the issues associated with measuring health gain are addressed in Chapter 7.

Measuring utility

One other example that makes healthcare and therefore the market for healthcare stand out, is that we do not just receive utility from our own personal consumption of healthcare or access to health services but also from the improved health of our family and friends. In addition, we also have the warm glow from just knowing that there is a healthcare system that will treat people if they need it.

PHARMACOECONOMICS

Pharmacoeconomics adopts and applies the principles and methodologies of health economics to the field of pharmaceuticals and pharmaceutical policy. Pharmacoeconomic evaluation therefore makes use of the broad range of techniques used in health economics evaluation to the specific context of medicines management. The aim of this book is to ensure that decision makers understand, as far as possible, this area of analysis.

Pharmacoeconomic evaluation is dominated by a simple theoretical concept: that of cost effectiveness. In general, we take the concept of cost effectiveness to imply either that we wish to achieve some predetermined objective at least cost or, alternatively, that we want to maximise the benefit to patients generated from a given limited amount of resources. To achieve this aim, we use the tools of economic evaluation to select the most efficient options from a range of healthcare alternatives to maximise the healthcare benefit of the population served. In addition, the increasingly stringent resource constraints imposed upon health services today require us to prioritise healthcare provision (i.e. we have to decide which healthcare programmes are most efficient, perhaps so that they can be provided first). Economic evaluation helps us prioritise services rationally by providing a scientific, value-free framework. This approach is very attractive to both government and healthcare decision makers. The remainder of this chapter provides an introduction to the four main methods of economic evaluation. Some examples are used to illustrate how it is used within the framework of pharmacoeconomics.

Issues in pharmacoeconomic evaluation

Perspective

Perspective is a key point to consider in any economic evaluation, that is, from whose point of view the study is conducted – the health service, where only direct costs are considered, or from a societal viewpoint where **indirect costs** are studied as well. In general, the societal perspective is considered the most appropriate but healthcare managers faced with a limited budget have a strong incentive to ignore the societal view and concentrate entirely on the costs that fall on their own budgets (Box 1.1).

Cost

The first distinction is that between financial and economic concepts of cost:

- Financial costs relate to monetary payments and usually reflect the price of a good or service.
- In economics, cost is concerned with a wider concept of resource use, including certain resources for which no monetary payment is made.

Thus, the time spent by patients in a hospital waiting room is a real cost to them. It is incurred during treatment but they receive no financial payment to cover this cost. The economic concept of cost is based on the realisation that the use of a resource in one way prevents it being used in alternative ways. Thus the true cost underlying a resource that is used in a particular manner is the benefits that are sacrificed from using the same resource in different ways. In economics, this true cost is known as the **opportunity cost**. Although in practice we do not measure opportunity cost, it is a very useful way of thinking because it helps us to make more informed decisions.

Opportunity cost. Opportunity cost can be defined as the 'benefit foregone when selecting one therapy alternative over the next best alternative'. What is

---

Box 1.1   Perspective in pharmacoeconomic evaluation

A study of different treatments for the relief of back pain, which considers costs imposed on only the health service, might suggest that treatment can be costly and is of limited benefit. By contrast, a study that takes a societal perspective would also incorporate the wider benefits arising to society, such as a reduction in working days lost and the patients' enhanced ability to undertake activities of daily living.

> **Concept box 1.9 – Opportunity cost**
>
> Economists perceive the true cost of any good or service in relation to the resources that are consumed to provide the good/service. The cost of the resources consumed is expressed as the value of the output that would arise through the next-best alternative use of the resources.

of concern to us is not how much a healthcare intervention costs but what we have to give up to use that intervention. This is a concept familiar to all of us, although perhaps not under this title. For instance, suppose I can afford to either buy a new car or to take an expensive holiday. The opportunity cost of buying a car is my inability to enjoy the benefits of taking a holiday.

Measuring costs. Several costs can be measured when weighing up the costs of any intervention. Which we choose to measure depends on whose perspective we decide to take and what kind of study we are interested in. These costs might be:

- *Direct:* paid directly by the health service, including staff costs, **capital costs**, drug **acquisition costs**.
- *Indirect:* costs experienced by the patient (or family or friends) or society. For example, these might include loss of earnings or loss of productivity. Many of these costs are difficult to measure but should be of concern to society as a whole.
- *Intangible:* these are the pain, worry or other distress that patients and/or their families suffer. These might be impossible to measure in monetary terms, or even at all, and so are not always considered in economic evaluations. Nevertheless, they are of concern to both doctors and patients.

Incremental analysis. When we evaluate healthcare interventions, we are always interested in both the costs and benefits of the intervention. We want to know how much it costs *and* how much more it costs than the current intervention; we want to know how many benefits it generates *and* how many more benefits it generates than the intervention we are currently using. When we talk about incremental analysis we are usually comparing costs and benefits between programmes.

This gives rise to a second, related concept of **marginal costs**. Marginal costs are the additional costs incurred when we increase our output within a healthcare programme. For instance, if a new treatment enables patients to be discharged from hospital a day earlier than they otherwise would be, it might be tempting to estimate the **average cost** of a hospital bed day as a saving of resources. But however this new treatment worked, all the fixed capital charges for a hospital bed – which go into the average cost, e.g. costs of laboratories, kitchens, and building maintenance – will be largely unchanged. The only costs that change will be those of having a patient physically occupy the bed – the costs of the patient's meals, treatment and perhaps nursing time. These are the marginal costs, where resource use is directly related to the

11

> ## Concept box 1.10 – Incremental or marginal costs
>
> These two concepts are frequently used interchangeably. However, incremental cost is more correctly applied to the difference in cost between healthcare programmes, whereas marginal cost shows how costs and benefits change if output is slightly increased or decreased within a healthcare programme. Marginal cost thus measures the cost of providing one additional unit of goods/services (e.g. one additional inpatient episode for a hip replacement patient).

change in the scale of service provision – the additional resource required to treat an additional patient or, conversely, the level of resource directly saved by treating one less patient.

METHODS OF ECONOMIC EVALUATION

Economic evaluation essentially provides us with a framework for drawing up a balance sheet of costs and benefits. It is this systematic and objective framework that helps decision makers to make more informed choices in their everyday working lives. All economic evaluations have a common structure in that they involve explicit measurement of inputs ('costs') and outcomes ('benefits') around medical interventions.

We've already looked at the way in which costs are treated in economic evaluation; we now turn our attention to how we can conceptualise and measure outcomes. The benefits we expect from an intervention might be measured in the following ways:

- *Natural units:* e.g. years of life saved, strokes prevented, ulcers healed.
- *Utility units:* the quality-adjusted life-year (QALY) is a widely used utility measure that combines quality and quantity of life in a single score.
- *Associated economic benefit:* this is usually measured in money, which is a useful common denominator allowing comparisons across different types of healthcare intervention. This measure includes, for instance, the economic benefits of an employee returning to work after illness.

The four main methods of economic evaluation are now described briefly; they are discussed in more detail in Chapter 7.

Cost minimisation analysis

In **cost minimisation analysis** (CMA), only the costs of the interventions under evaluation are measured. The perspective is usually that of the health service; CMA can be only used when the health benefits of the healthcare treatments are identical and therefore need not be considered separately. An example would be a decision to prescribe a generic drug instead of a brand

> **Concept box 1.11 – Structures of economic evaluation**
>
> | | |
> |---|---|
> | Cost minimisation analysis (CMA) | Benefits assumed to be equivalent |
> | Cost effectiveness analysis (CEA) | Benefits measured in natural units |
> | Cost utility analysis (CUA) | Benefits measured in terms of 'utility' (e.g. QALY) |
> | Cost benefit analysis (CBA) | Benefits reduced to their financial equivalent |

name drug, which should, in theory, achieve the same effect at less cost. This form of evaluation cannot be used to consider different programmes or therapies with different outcomes.

Cost effectiveness analysis

The term 'cost effectiveness' properly refers to an evaluation where the health benefit can be defined and measured in natural units (e.g. years of life saved, ulcers healed). **Cost effectiveness analysis** (CEA) compares therapies whose outcomes can be measured in the same natural units and measures costs in money. For instance, if our desired outcome was relief of severe reflux oesophagitis, we could consider the costs per patient relieved of symptoms using a proton pump inhibitor compared to those using H_2 blockers. CEA is the most commonly applied form of economic analysis in the health economics literature and is often used in drug therapy. It does not allow comparisons to be made between two totally different areas of medicine with different outcomes.

Cost utility analysis

Cost utility analysis (CUA) is similar to cost effectiveness analysis in that there is a defined outcome and the cost to reach that outcome is measured in money. However, here the outcome of interest is a unit of utility (e.g. a QALY; see Concept box 1.12, p. 14). Because the endpoint might not be directly dependent on the disease state, CUA can, in theory, look at more than one area of medicine (e.g. cost per QALY of coronary artery bypass grafting versus cost per QALY in using erythropoietin in renal disease). In practice, this is not so easy because the QALY is subject to much philosophical and technical criticism. The usefulness of the QALY is debated in Chapter 7.

Cost benefit analysis

Here, the benefit is measured as the associated economic benefit of an intervention, and hence both costs and benefits are expressed in money. **Cost benefit analysis** (CBA) can ignore many intangible but very important

> **Concept box 1.12 – Quality-adjusted life-year (QALY)**
>
> The concept of the QALY is based on the belief that the aim of any healthcare intervention can be dichotomised between improving survival (increasing the quantity of life) and improving the ability to enjoy life (enhancing quality of life). By applying 'quality weights' to each additional year of life experienced after treatment, the QALY attempts to incorporate both of these elements into a single measure.

benefits, which are difficult to measure in money terms (e.g. relief of anxiety). CBA can also seem to discriminate against those in whom a return to productive employment is unlikely (e.g. the elderly or the unemployed). However, the virtue of this analysis is that it allows comparisons between very different areas, and not only advances within the field of medicine. For example, using CBA, the costs and benefits of expanding university education (benefits of improved education and hence productivity) can be compared to establishing a back pain service (enhancing productivity by returning patients to work). This approach is not widely accepted for use in health economics.

Cost consequences and other types of evaluation

Other forms of evaluation that consider costs and benefits to some extent are to be found in the literature. In some cases, often where studies consider multiple outcomes, costs and benefits are presented in a disaggregated form (e.g. health profiles). These evaluations are frequently referred to as cost consequences analyses. **Burden of disease** (also known as cost of illness) studies attempt to measure the health and resource implications arising to society from a particular disease. Although such studies might help to generate useful descriptive data, they are of limited value in informing healthcare decision making. In particular, they do not consider the availability of effective interventions aimed at reducing this measured burden of disease. For further discussion of such issues, see Chapter 6.

DISCOUNTING

There is often a difference in timing between the investment of health-service resources and the associated health gain. In general, we prefer to receive benefits now and pay costs in the future. To reflect this in economic evaluation, costs are **discounted**; the current discount rate set by the UK Treasury is 6%. There is some debate over whether benefits should also be discounted. It is relatively easy to accept that £100 spent now is worth more now than it will be in 5 years time but how does one compare a healthy year now to a healthy year in 5 years time? In health economics, the rate most commonly used to discount benefits is 1.5%, as recommended by the National Institute for Clinical Excellence (NICE).

UNCERTAINTY

Economics operates in the realm of the behavioural sciences and, as such, is beset by uncertainty. Any estimate of costs and benefits will therefore also be affected by uncertainty concerning the exact values of such costs and benefits. There will also be areas where clinical evidence is either limited or entirely missing. When conducting a pharmacoeconomic analysis it is therefore often necessary to make assumptions to supplement the structure of evidence obtained from clinical trials and other sources. All pharmacoeconomic analyses must therefore include a **sensitivity analysis** to assess the robustness of the study results in relation to variations in the certainty of the assumptions made. Sensitivity analysis can be used to assess the robustness of the results of any economic analysis. The economic appraisal can be said to be robust if the results are not influenced to any great extent by feasible variations in the exact value of any of the key underlying assumptions.

Identifying changes in resource use in economic evaluations can be likened to dropping a stone into the middle of a millpond. For example, take the example of the apparently simple effects of the introduction of a short-acting anaesthetic such as propafol – these drugs have revolutionised much of surgical practice by allowing a shift to day-case surgery. The immediate and most visible surrounding ripples will affect resource use in the surgical directorate (Fig. 1.3). Further (but more 'dampened' ripples) will affect the pharmacy as a consequence of the enhanced cost of short-acting anaesthetics. Further out will be changes in demand for hotel services in the hospital (laundry, catering, etc.) as a consequence of reduced lengths of hospital stay. Many of the ripples outside the immediate epicentre of the change will also affect the primary healthcare sector (increased demand for GP consultations and community care services), other public services (short-term provision of a home help or meals on wheels) and privately borne costs (increased burden of care at home). The ripples emanating from the centre of the change are potentially endless, but become less significant as the distance from the centre increases. This example illustrates the difficulty encountered in identifying all changes in resource use that can occur in health economic evaluations. The extent to which analyses need to incorporate resource ripples as they move further from the epicentre of the change depends largely on the perspective from which the analysis is undertaken.

Concept box 1.13 – Sensitivity analysis

In sensitivity analyses, different assumptions are substituted into the evaluation to test whether the study results are robust or if they can be influenced by the substitution.

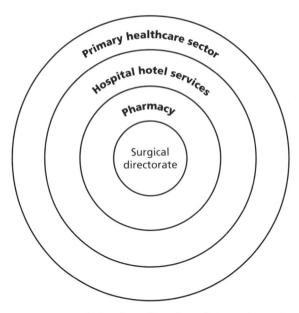

Fig 1.3 Changing resources: the knock-on effect of introducing a short-acting anaesthetic in surgery

Conclusion

This chapter has examined the principles and practice underlying health economics analyses. It has emphasised that the use of health economics methods is a valuable tool for improving the information base upon which healthcare decisions are made. We have stressed that health economics can be considered a tool that can help to inform and improve decision making, rather than a device for actually making decisions. In many ways, its value is as a systematic and objective system of thought. The very process of identifying alternative options to meet prespecified objectives and balancing resources and benefits represents a valuable mode of thinking for decision making, irrespective of whether a formal economic appraisal has been undertaken.

This chapter has also introduced the manner in which these principles are applied in health economic evaluations by exploring the nature and application of economic evaluation techniques. Further explanation of these techniques is presented in Chapter 7. At the end of this book, a glossary of terms has been provided with the aim of further demystifying the jargon that is frequently used in the areas of health economics and pharmacoeconomics.

Health economics is not inherently difficult to understand. Its simple premise is that decision making concerning healthcare choices should be based upon the evaluation and comparison of both the costs and benefits arising from all the therapeutic options available, and that the best decision making requires a sensitive balance of both of these dimensions. How this can be achieved in practice is illustrated in detail in the rest of this book.

The economics of healthcare and healthcare systems

2

INTRODUCTION

What are health systems and what are their goals? How do these relate to economics? This is important in trying to understand the context within which **health economics** – and specifically **pharmacoeconomics** – operates, and this chapter tries to answer some of these questions. In addition, it explains the different ways in which health systems are funded and examines the incentives and constraints operating on clinical decision makers under different types of healthcare system.

WHAT ARE HEALTHCARE SYSTEMS AND WHAT ARE THEIR GOALS?

The World Health Organization (WHO 2001) defines a health system as:

> … comprising all the organisations, institutions and resources that are devoted to producing health actions. A health action is defined as any effort, whether in personal healthcare, public health services, or through intersectoral initiatives whose primary purpose is to improve health.

This means that although factors such as housing, income and education all contribute greatly to health status, they would be excluded from the definition because their primary purpose is not a health action. Although health economists recognise that factors outside the healthcare system have a great influence on health, health economic evaluations tend to concentrate on those health actions within healthcare systems. This is in part because the funders of economic evaluation are often concerned with the healthcare budget and not, for example, with the housing or education budget. (This issue of perspective will be discussed in more detail in Chapter 7.) In addition, measuring health outcomes associated with improved housing or additional educational resources is very difficult because the cause-and-effect relationships are complex, likely to occur over a long period of time and therefore hard to delineate.

Health actions, or the desire to improve health, are certainly central features of healthcare systems (Box 2.1). However, the improvement of health is not

---

Box 2.1   Aims of a health service

- Improve public and individual health
- Treat individual sick
- Promote solidarity
- Maximise the number of patients treated
- Maximise quality of treatment
- Be efficient
- Achieve some mix of all of the above objectives.

---

the only goal operating here. In addition, most healthcare systems aim to limit the financial burdens of ill health so that treatment is not totally dependent on one's ability to pay, and to respond to people's expectations of the system. This latter goal is important because people might expect the system to support heroic or expensive attempts to save the lives of patients whose chance of survival is extremely limited or non-existent. On health economic grounds, such attempts would be deemed a poor use of resources but this so-called 'rule of rescue' commands public support and cannot be ignored.

Expectations are in part a product of government policies and pronouncements. When governments promise minimum standards of care or quality improvements, public expectations of the system are raised. For example, in the UK the National Service Frameworks define appropriate standards for managing certain conditions. But, in turn, expectations also influence government policy. For this reason, some of the actions produced by the healthcare system might be geared to providing symbolic reassurance in the form of highly visible, rather than cost effective, care. This in part explains why, in many healthcare systems, we might observe features like the maintenance of small and costly – but popular – local hospitals, the provision of immediate-access walk-in clinics despite the lack of evidence for their **effectiveness**, and the avoidance of explicit **rationing**.

Healthcare systems aim to deliver health actions by using resources efficiently and in a manner that promotes **equity** in healthcare. However, although rising expectations about the ability of healthcare systems to deliver can act as an impetus for continuous improvements in care, these expectations can also act to undermine the equity and efficiency aims of the system. As we have discussed, pursuing the rule of rescue might result in an inefficient allocation of resources. Similarly, some sections of the public might see certain types of patient or disease (e.g. children or cancer sufferers) as more worthy of healthcare resources than others (e.g. drug abusers or people with HIV/Aids).

Concept box 2.1 – Equity

Equity refers to a desire to share benefits and cost fairly across the community. But it can have many different definitions and what is fair is debated.

Box 2.2   Efficiency and equity (from Ubel et al 1996)

Would you sacrifice efficiency for equity? Look at the example below and make your choice.

You have a fixed budget of $200 000 and, as a decision maker, you are faced with a choice between two screening tests for colon cancer in a population at low risk. The tests have different costs and sensitivity/specificity:

- Test 1 would cost $200 000 to screen the whole population and would prevent 1000 deaths
- Test 2 would cost $400,000 to screen the whole population and would prevent 2200 deaths. This means that only half of the population can be screened for your budget of $200 000
- Test 2 saves 100 more lives (i.e. 1100 – 1000) but screens only half of the population.

Would you choose to screen all with test 1 or screen half and save more lives with test 2? In this scenario, three types of people were asked to choose between the two cancer-screening tests: members of the public, ethicists and medical decision makers.

On analysis, 56% of the members of the public and 53% of the ethicists were in favour of test 1, which screened everyone but saved fewer lives. However, the majority (56%) of the decision makers were in favour of test 2. But it is worth remembering that this was a hypothetical example. How easy would it be in the real world for decision makers to pursue a policy of screening only half of the population? How would they select that half and how acceptable would this be to the population as a whole?

When it comes to equity and efficiency in healthcare systems, there might be a trade-off between the two. There is much evidence to suggest that members of the public would sacrifice efficiency to some extent to achieve greater equity in the system (Box 2.2).

WHAT DOES EQUITY MEAN IN THE CONTEXT OF HEALTHCARE SYSTEMS?

In the example in Box 2.2, equity means treating everybody the same, in the sense that they all have an equal opportunity of being screened if test 1 is chosen. It is important to note, however, that although most people see equity in healthcare as important, there is much less consensus about what the term 'equity' actually means. Measuring the extent to which healthcare systems achieve equity is also a contentious issue. Some argue that that there can be no right or wrong definition of equity, and that it is independent of some view of what society or healthcare is about and to what extent it wishes to redistribute wealth or other benefits. Once this is clear, then it is possible to judge statements about equity in terms of the extent to which they are consistent or inconsistent with these goals.

In making judgements about what is equitable, we might try to frame a judgement so that it is made independently of the interests of the person making it. The decision makers might be placed behind a 'veil of ignorance' such that they do not know what their own position in society would be. As the individual making the judgement does not know whether they would be poor or rich, they are likely to choose a society that gives greatest advantage to the worst-off members.

However, there are problems with this approach. For one thing if we adopt policies that improve things for the worst-off members of society, then we now create a new but different group of people who are the worst-off. Another problem is the extent to which, in practice, people who already have a place in society can put that to one side and make judgements *as if* they do not know their place in society. As we discussed earlier, funders of economic evaluation might be interested only in those costs which relate to the budgets for which they have responsibility. Similarly, the views of **stakeholders** in relation to healthcare will depend on their position within the system. Different individuals will adopt different **perspectives**. For example, a new drug, which is cost effective and produces savings in the long-term but results in increased expenditure in the short-term, might present a problem to somebody who is responsible for balancing the annual budget. For individual clinicians or patients, however, the preference might be to invest in this drug now and take the resources from somewhere (anywhere, but 'not from my backyard') else in the system.

It is even more complicated than just different stakeholders having different perspectives, because the *same* individual might adopt *different* perspectives depending on the decision-making context. For example, an individual taxpayer might not support the use of high-cost drugs that have limited **efficacy**, but if they or a member of their family become ill and these drugs offer some hope, then they might support the use of these drugs. Posing the question in terms of population health gain or statistical lives can produce very different answers from those received when the choice is about identified patients, particularly when these patients are known to the respondent.

Equity in healthcare is a complicated business. However, we might be able to reach agreement on some things. For example if, as in the example in Box 2.2, we are faced with a group of people with similar characteristics in terms of their risk of cancer, we might want to treat them all the same. However, if we had a group of high-risk patients and a group of low-risk patients, we might prioritise the high-risk group in terms of the screening or treatment programme – on the grounds that this is where we will get the greatest return on our investment. Economic evaluation can be a very useful tool in identifying this (Box 2.3).

So we might agree that people who are alike in relevant respects should be treated alike, and that people who are different in relevant respects should be

---

Box 2.3   Who to treat?

Lowering cholesterol reduces the risk of heart attacks by about 30%. But whom should we treat with expensive cholesterol-lowering drugs? From a public health perspective, we should target therapy to those with the greatest risk of heart attack (i.e. patients with a previous heart attack, who have a high risk of 8% per year of a further heart attack) rather than at patients with just a slightly high cholesterol and no other risk factors, whose risk of a heart attack is about 1% per year. The reasoning is that treating each will cost the same but the benefits are greater for the high-risk patient (30% of 8% is more than 30% of 1%). This is government policy in the UK in this area.

But individual patients might feel differently about this – a low-risk patient might argue that he or she is as entitled to treatment as anyone else!

treated in proportion to that difference. The 'relevant respect' in this example is risk of cancer, and this helps us to prioritise treatment or investigation.

Are there other relevant aspects we might consider? The number of possible options include:

- **willingness to pay** for care
- current health status
- expenditure equality
- capacity to benefit
- resources required to exceed **capacity to benefit**
- entitlement to equal health.

Willingness to pay (WTP) for care. If the aim of a healthcare system is to maximise social welfare, then those who value healthcare most should receive treatment. One way to evaluate who values healthcare most is to investigate which patients would be most willing to pay for it and how much they would be willing to pay. As a method, willingness to pay is flawed in health services that are traditionally free at point of delivery, and it might not work well in those where the patient knows the bill is picked up by a third-party payer. It is also difficult to disentangle willingness to pay from ability to pay, so this might favour the rich over the poor. This method used in economic evaluation is discussed more in Chapter 7.

Current health status. Under this argument, people with pneumonia receive treatment before people with a common cold. However, people who are severely ill and beyond hope (remember the rule of rescue!) will be prioritised over others whose prospects for health gain are much greater. This is often the most socially and medically acceptable way to select patients for treatment, regardless of the inefficiency.

Equality of expenditure. The idea here is that as citizens we each have an equal and finite allowance in terms of resources available for healthcare. This might provide an incentive to adopt a healthy lifestyle but it ignores the fact that ill health is unequally distributed in society and that **average costs** (and allowance) would go little way towards treating the cost of a single serious episode – so what would you do when your share of the budget is spent? Or if you were well and never spent any of your budget?

Capacity to benefit. Rather than prioritising treatment on the basis of severity of illness, most health economists would advocate that treatment should be based on an individual's capacity to benefit from treatment. This is aimed at ensuring that the maximum health gain is secured from limited healthcare resources.

As we have seen, whereas economists are concerned with efficiency (i.e. obtaining the most from limited resources), healthcare systems pursue several goals, of which health improvement is only one. Adopting a capacity to benefit approach to healthcare delivery might mean treating more affluent patients on the grounds that the lifestyles associated with their higher incomes will allow them to benefit more from treatment than those on low incomes living in damp housing and with poor diets. We might favour young patients with a potentially longer life expectancy over older patients, or ignore the most seriously ill (who will probably die whatever we do) in favour of the less seriously ill.

This would conflict with the equity goals of the system. Similarly, capacity to benefit might result in the prioritisation of chiropody services over intensive care units. This would undermine the ability of healthcare systems to provide reassurance and respond to public expectations.

Entitlement to equal health. Here, the emphasis is on the outcome of the process as opposed to resource inputs. The idea of equal health is a Utopian notion and is unlikely to be achieved in practice, although it could be argued that healthcare systems should have this as their (albeit idealistic) goal because what matters ultimately is health status and not the inputs in terms of individual services. However, we should not lose sight of the fact that processes – as well as outcomes – are important to individuals. Indeed, one of the areas on which the WHO assesses the performance of healthcare systems concerns the way in which patients are treated (in terms of factors such as dignity, autonomy, confidentiality, prompt attention) within the healthcare system.

We should also remember that equity applies to the financing of care as well as to its delivery. The next section ('Market failure, third-party payment and healthcare systems', p. 24) examines the equity and efficiency consequences of various methods for financing healthcare and explains why it is that leaving healthcare to the free market is unlikely to produce an optimal allocation of healthcare resources.

Evaluating healthcare systems

Given the conflicting goals, not always explicitly stated, one might wonder how one would ever evaluate a healthcare system. One way is if the health service has set itself any targets – for instance, the target in the UK NHS is that 75% of patients with myocardial infarction will receive potentially life-saving thrombolysis within 20 minutes of entering the hospital. In practice, there are relatively few targets common to several health services and, although they are useful benchmarks within a service, they do not enable comparisons to be drawn with other systems.

The World Health Organization made a bold attempt to compare national health services in 2000. It did this by examining national health services under different domains, including health outcomes (a basket of morbidity and mortality indicators), expenditure per head of population, fairness of financial contribution, efficiency and responsiveness in terms of respecting people's dignity and autonomy.

These measures, and how they are made, are highly controversial and have been heavily criticised; they should not be accepted uncritically. But whatever its flaws, the results of the WHO report are interesting (Table 2.1). The report argues that the quality of a health service might depend less on the resources it has to spend and more on how they are spent (Box 2.4).

So it might matter less how much you spend than what you spend it on. Whereas the US scores highly on responsiveness amongst those receiving

Table 2.1 National rankings for health indicators (WHO 2001)

Country	Health spend per capita rank	Performance	
		Level of health rank	Overall system ranking
Australia	17	39	32
Austria	6	15	9
Canada	10	35	30
France	4	4	1
Germany	3	41	25
Greece	30	11	14
Ireland	25	32	19
Italy	11	3	2
Japan	13	9	10
Netherlands	9	19	17
New Zealand	20	80	41
Sweden	7	21	23
Turkey	82	33	70
UK	26	24	18
United States	1	72	37

Box 2.4   WHO report (2001) – health outcomes and spending

'If Sweden enjoys better health than Uganda – life expectancy is almost twice as long – that is in large part because it spends exactly 35 times as much per capita on its health system. But Pakistan spends almost precisely the same amount per person as Uganda, out of an income per person that is close to Uganda's, and yet it has a life expectancy almost 25 years higher. This is the crucial comparison: why are health outcomes in Pakistan so much better, for the same expenditure?

treatment (ranked number 1 worldwide), the American emphasis on insurance-based funding, covered mainly by employers, and a minimal safety net cover means that many Americans have no medical cover at all. This accounts in part for the poor (relative to expenditure) showing of the US on health performance (ranking 72). In addition, the US system has higher administrative **overheads** than the UK NHS because of the volume of paperwork required to support billing and **reimbursement** of care in the insurance-based system.

If we look at rates of healthcare consumption by **gross domestic product** (GDP) rather than by actual spend as in the WHO figures, it is clear that the UK devotes a lower proportion of its GDP to healthcare than most other OECD countries (Table 2.2). The question of whether, for instance, the UK, with one

Table 2.2   Spending on healthcare – international comparisons (OECD 2000)

Country	Per cent GDP 1997
EU15 average	7.9
Australia	8.3
Austria	7.9
Canada	9.3
France	9.9
Germany	10.4
Greece	7.1
Ireland	7.0
Italy	7.6
Japan	7.3
Netherlands	8.5
New Zealand	7.6
Sweden	8.6
Turkey	4.6
UK	6.7
USA	14.0

of the lower spends, should spend more is not a question for health economists but for politicians – as it is in all states with a universalist healthcare system.

So the question of how much should be spent in a health service is difficult and international comparisons – so beloved of politicians – need to be interpreted very carefully.

MARKET FAILURE, THIRD-PARTY PAYMENT AND HEALTHCARE SYSTEMS

Whereas many goods and services are bought and sold using market mechanisms, health economists agree that particular characteristics associated with healthcare make it unsuited to exchange in a free market. We would expect attempts at pure market exchange to result in market failure for a number of reasons. These are the:

- unpredictable nature of demand and associated risk in relation to healthcare and illness
- existence of externalities
- asymmetrical distribution of information between those who consume and those who supply care.

Unpredictable demand and associated financial risk

Whereas we can plan our consumption of goods such as bread and butter, we cannot do the same for our future consumption of healthcare because the onset of illness is often unpredictable. Where care is left to the free market, we expect insurance companies to offer health cover to individuals in return for the payment of premiums. The costs to the company will be the fixed costs of running their business together with some element of profit and healthcare expenditures paid out for insured clients. These costs will be reflected in the premiums charged. This means that if everybody faces the same risk of illness, the charges to the individual over time will be greater than their expected expenditure on healthcare. However, because the insurance company takes away the element of risk, many people will be content to pay the premiums. This all works fine in theory but in practice there are a number of reasons why this would not work in a health service and why market forces would fail here. Before reviewing these, it is important to note that a free market is not the same as a service designed around social insurance (where everyone must join and there is no loading of premiums for risk), or in insurance that is a supplement to some other funded health service. These reasons are:

- diseconomies of scale
- **adverse selection**
- moral hazard.

Diseconomies of scale

For any insurance company, there will be certain fixed costs, which do not vary with the scale of its operations. These might include advertising expenses or the cost of a secretary for the managing director. The larger a firm gets, the more units (here the units would be insurance policies) it has over which to spread these fixed costs. This means that premiums will be cheaper with larger firms. Competition in the market means lots of small firms offering premiums and all incurring fixed costs. The unit cost of premiums in such a market is likely therefore to be high and represents an inefficient use of resources because fewer larger-scale firms could reduce unit costs. In theory, costs would be lowest with just one large company benefiting from economies of scale. However, in practice the absence of competition could lead this company to exploit its monopoly power and charge high prices.

Diseconomies of scale can result in market failure because people would prefer to pay for care via a publicly funded tax-based system that costs them less than paying high premiums brought on by large numbers of competitive firms or an exploitative monopoly provider.

Adverse selection

In a competitive market for health insurance, companies might have no idea of the risk status of an individual. Premiums would therefore have to be set based on the general risk of the insured population. The premium paid would be the same for everybody who takes out insurance. However, whereas the company has no knowledge of risk status, individuals are rather better informed on the matter. For those who perceive themselves to be below average risk, the average premium could be perceived as being too high and they might withdraw from the scheme. This leaves a group of uninsured low-risk individuals and could encourage the development of policies tailored to the individual in response to this market opportunity. This process of selecting out the lowest-risk groups is called 'adverse selection'. However, because insurers might not have access to information on which to discriminate between low- and high-risk patients, they might refuse to offer such policies.

When low-risk groups leave the scheme, the average risk for those remaining increases. This means that expected healthcare expenditures and, as a result, premiums would be higher for those remaining. Because in general the health of the poor is worse than that of the more affluent members of society, the higher-risk groups will typically include people on low incomes, who might not be able to afford to pay the higher premiums.

Adverse selection leads to market failure because the low-risk patients are willing to buy insurance paying a premium based on their level of risk, but asymmetry of information means that companies are unwilling to provide such cover. In addition, a large number of people on low incomes will be uninsured because they are unable to afford to pay a fair premium that reflects their relatively high-risk status.

Moral hazard

Moral hazard refers to the phenomenon in insurance-based systems whereby levels of demand for and supply of healthcare are greater than they would be if fully informed individuals bought healthcare in a perfectly competitive market. This inflated demand and supply arises because insurance reduces the costs of care to consumers, which means they have less incentive to adopt a healthy lifestyle. In addition, because the cost of care at the point of delivery

---

Concept box 2.2 – Third-party payment and the problem of moral hazard

Third-party payment arises from a pooling of risk in healthcare – we pay taxes or premiums so that, when we are ill, we are cushioned from some of the effects of illness and I, personally (first party), do not have to pay the doctor (second party) who is instead paid by the state or insurance (third party). So my ability to pay at the time of illness does not determine whether I can receive treatment. However, this gives rise to **moral hazard** – a temptation for the first party to consume more than is strictly needed (like inflating an insurance claim) or for the second party to provide more than is strictly needed.

is nil to the consumer, there are incentives to consume more care than would otherwise be the case.

In addition to this **'consumer moral hazard'** there is also 'provider moral hazard', often termed **'supplier-induced demand'**. The idea here is that doctors will induce demand, providing more care than would otherwise be the case. The patient is happy to acquiesce in such circumstances because the cost of care is covered by health insurance.

Moral hazard is a feature of healthcare systems that do not rely solely on direct payment for care; it is discussed in more detail below.

Externalities

'Externalities' are spillover effects from other people's consumption of healthcare. In addition to any direct impact on the individual consumer there are other wider effects, which can be favourable or unfavourable. For example, we get benefits from a vaccination programme that others have participated in. This 'selfish externality' occurs when we get a direct benefit – in terms of our reduced likelihood of contracting disease – because a vaccination programme will reduce the number of carriers (and hence our personal risk of disease).

We also get benefits from knowing that those who need healthcare are able to get it (i.e. a 'caring externality'). If individuals pay directly for care, the market price is unlikely to reflect the additional benefits (positive externalities) of the care. People might be willing to pay only for what they perceive as their own personal benefits and not for the wider societal benefits (i.e. the externalities). This could result in the underproduction of healthcare viewed from a societal perspective. In other words, a pure market for healthcare based on individual purchases might not serve societal welfare.

Asymmetry of information

When we are ill, we often do not know what ails us. Similarly, although we want to get well, we are often not sure what will make us well because we are unlikely to be fully informed about the range of available healthcare treatments that could benefit us. This asymmetry of information between providers and consumers of care means that individuals are reliant on the advice of suppliers of care, who act as agents on their behalf. Ideally, patients want their doctor to act as a 'perfect agent' on their behalf. This would entail the doctor putting his or her own interests to one side and objectively supplying information to patients, who can then make a fully informed decision maximising their own **utility**. However, doctors might not always act in patients' best interest; this is explored further in the 'Incentives and supplier-induced demand', p. 31.

Third-party payment in healthcare systems

Healthcare systems reflect the underlying values and the historical and socioeconomic context of the country in which they are situated. In this sense, no two healthcare systems are the same. However, in the developed world, what all of these systems have in common is that they embody some form of third-party payment. This means that financing of care is separated from the consumption of care, with a third party paying some or all of the costs of care. Hence, in the UK the NHS is 'free at the point of delivery', although citizens pay for it elsewhere.

The third party might be government, as in the UK and for Medicare and Medicaid patients (the poor and the elderly) in the US. Alternatively, the payment might be made by a social insurance fund, as is the case in Germany. Here payments are made to the funds by means of an obligatory payroll tax. Private insurance is another form of third-party payment that accounts for 10% of health expenditure in the UK and 50% in the US.

By contrast, many developing countries are characterised by out-of-pocket payment systems. Here healthcare is treated as just another commodity in the marketplace and government's role is usually small or non-existent. The problem with this type of arrangement is that often those in need are least able to pay and this is exacerbated as poor health reduces an individual's ability to earn.

The rationale for third-party payment

The problems associated with out-of-pocket payment systems explain why third-party payment as a means of financing care has developed in Western economies. There are issues of social solidarity as well as a recognition that healthcare is too important to be left to the market. The rationale for third-party payment depends partly on the perspective adopted by those who comment on the subject.

For health economists, third-party payment is a response to market failure for the reasons we have discussed above.

Another explanation for third-party payment is that in modern industrialised societies such systems developed in response to the needs of an educated and enfranchised workforce and are symptomatic of a growing political commitment to equity. An alternative view – and one that is often illustrated by reference to the US healthcare system – is that provider interest groups encouraged the growth of third-party payment. At its most cynical, this means that doctors are better paid when the patient doesn't have to worry about paying the doctor directly, and so are encouraged to consume more healthcare, or that insurance and pharmaceutical companies have a vested interest in the growth of the market for healthcare insurance. If this is true, then these powerful vested interests might be able to resist healthcare reform despite economic arguments in its favour.

Equity and efficiency consequences of third-party payment

There are many ways of providing third-party payment health systems. These schemes are not 'neutral', or merely a technical response to the issue of providing healthcare, but embody deeply political issues. The values underlying schemes vary enormously, as can be seen in the extent to which risks are pooled.

Tax-based systems, such as in the UK, pool the risks across a whole population and spread the risk most equitably. In the US the notion of government taking responsibility for raising taxes to fund healthcare and ensuring the provision of care for all citizens has been resisted on the grounds that such 'nanny state' behaviour would represent an unacceptable infringement of individual liberty. Instead, individuals are free to choose whether to enter into some form of insurance arrangement for their healthcare. However, in the US an estimated one-sixth of the population is without insurance cover and the equity implications of these arrangements are unpalatable to those who see free healthcare as a basic right of citizenship. There are limited safety nets in the form of Medicare for the elderly (but no medicines coverage) and Medicaid for the poor, in addition to these insurance-based systems.

Most people in the UK regard healthcare as a basic entitlement of the citizen: 82% of Britons say that government should definitely be responsible for healthcare compared with 51% in Germany and 71% in Sweden (Fig. 2.1). Much lower levels of support are likely to be observed in the US.

Private insurance. Private insurance is unlikely to be concerned with equity: it will exclude high-risk populations (i.e. poorer sicker people, who would cost more than the premiums collected). In addition, private health insurance does not fare well in terms of efficiency because the administrative expenses associated with such systems are high, because of the need to assess risk, set premiums, design complex benefit schedules and review, pay or challenge claims.

Another problem with private insurance is that spending in such systems tends to be demand led, and commissioning fragmented, which results in increased costs overall. However, a positive aspect of this type of system is that, for those who can afford health insurance, choice and responsiveness are likely to be greater.

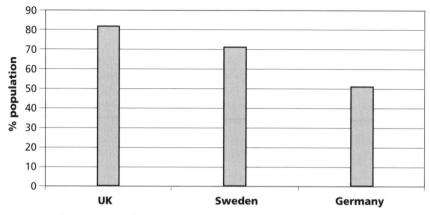

Fig 2.1 The percentage of the population who agree that government should be responsible for healthcare. From Jowell et al 1998.

General taxation. A tax-based system is universalist and redistributive because it tries to compensate in part for social inequalities. This means that government action encourages participation by individuals in society, and the notion of citizenship here includes the idea of social rights such as access to free healthcare; private insurance-based schemes imply a much narrower notion of citizenship. Tax-based schemes are more efficient than private insurance in the sense that the costs of administration are lower. The Wanless report (2001) on funding the UK NHS comments that:

> ... general taxation is widely regarded as being highly efficient from a macroeconomic perspective, delivering strong **cost containment** and forcing prioritisation through what are typically cash-limited healthcare budgets set by government. Under tax financing, the government has both a strong incentive and capacity to control costs.

However, many have argued that control of expenditure in the UK system has gone too far because of a reluctance to increase taxes. This, it is argued, has led to underinvestment over many years in the UK health service in comparison with other countries.

The funding of health services from general taxation means that the question of how much to spend on health services, as opposed to – say – defence or education, is largely a political decision based on the competing priorities of governments. This means that people who would be willing to pay more tax to fund healthcare are reluctant to pay more in general taxation because there are no guarantees that the extra revenue would be spent on health. Proponents of hypothecated taxation (i.e. a tax specifically for one purpose) argue that hypothecation would resolve this problem. One of the problems with hypothecation is that in times of recession, the tax yield might be low leaving a gap between projected demand and resources available. However, this is a potential problem for taxation-based schemes generally. It is also worth noting, however, that hypothecation reduces the choices available to civil servants and ministers in the Treasury, and this might also be a source of resistance to hypothecation.

A final point to note about funding from general taxation is that although it is likely to be more equitable and efficient than private insurance, it is likely to offer less choice to individuals.

Social insurance. In social insurance schemes, employer and/or employee earnings-related contributions are usually paid to social insurance or sickness funds. One criticism of this system is that the sickness funds that manage these payments have little incentive to contain costs because of their ability to raise contributions. The existence in some countries of multiple funds, and the resulting fragmentation in healthcare purchasing, can result in higher costs of administering the system. Furthermore, the experience in many European countries is that such schemes have had to be bailed out of financial difficulties by a central government drawing on central taxation.

These schemes can also be universalist and redistributive. The extent to which social insurance schemes are equitable depends on the nature of the particular system in operation. As with tax-based schemes, access to care does

The economics of healthcare and healthcare systems

not depend on ability to pay. The extent to which contributions reflect ability to pay does vary however, between different countries. They might also be less efficient than tax-based systems because the machinery to collect contributions and pay the bills from providers of healthcare can be cumbersome and expensive.

Although insurance schemes in theory help contain costs within the limits of the fund, in practice countries such as France and Germany are reforming healthcare because of the inability of funds to meet demand. France's social insurance contributions were seen as increasing the costs of labour and adversely affecting employment levels. Since 1998, employees' contributions have been largely replaced by an earmarked tax for health. Policies to contain costs by limiting payments provided by health insurance (e.g. fixing doctors' fees and halving the reimbursement level for gastroscopy) have also followed both in France and in Germany. In Germany these have prompted doctors to take strike action in protest.

Despite the many different ways of funding healthcare used across the globe, a common theme is the inability of health systems to keep pace with rising consumer expectations and technological advance. Cost containment in health is high on government agendas in both tax- and insurance-based systems.

A further criticism of occupationally related insurance schemes, whether social or private, is that they might give rise to 'job lock'. This means that worker mobility will be reduced because individuals whose employers provide health insurance as part of their employment package will be reluctant to move because they fear losing their insurance cover.

Unintended consequences of third-party payment systems

'Moral hazard' (see Concept box 2.2, p. 26) is a feature of third-party payment systems. This term is used to refer to inflated demand for or supply of healthcare. Because payment is separated from consumption, consumers do not face incentives to limit their consumption of care in the same way they would with direct payment. There is a danger, therefore, that third-party payment might lead to an inflated demand for care. This is known as 'consumer moral hazard'.

Because clinicians act as an agent for the patient and at the same time as a supplier of care, they might be inclined to induce demand ('**producer moral hazard**', more commonly known as 'supplier-induced demand') for their services. For example, a clinician who is paid on a fee-per-service basis might choose to undertake diagnostic tests such as endoscopy as first-line treatment for dyspepsia for young patients with no 'alarm' symptoms. This leads to a greater volume of care being demanded than would be the case under direct payment.

Incentives and supplier-induced demand

There are many ways of paying providers within healthcare systems. As we will see, each of these creates different incentives in relation to the supply of healthcare.

Fee-for-service. Under this system, doctors are paid a fee for each item of service they provide. The greater the number of items provided, the more the doctor is paid. Fee-for-service is often associated with supplier-induced demand because it creates financial incentives to provide inflated service levels.

Capitation. Capitation is used as a method of payment for GPs in the UK, where it represents around 60% of the income of an average GP. GPs are paid an amount for each person on their list, regardless of the level of care provided. One of the disadvantages of such an arrangement is that GPs might select-out patients who represent a high workload. In addition, capitation payments mean that there are no incentives to work harder because extra efforts are not rewarded. In theory, capitation encourages GPs to compete for patients, with hard-working, efficient practices attracting greater numbers of patients. However, the reasons why people choose their GP are many and varied, suggesting that the end result will not necessarily be increased efficiency in the provision of care.

Salaries. Here, clinician remuneration is not related to the volume of procedures performed or services provided. There are fewer incentives to inflate demand than with fee-for-service but guaranteeing doctors an income might reduce their incentive to work harder. In the UK, some GPs have expressed opposition to the introduction of salaried GP schemes on the grounds that GPs with no financial stake in a practice would be more likely to move around during their career, leading to a reduction in continuity of care. In addition, salaried doctors – because their income is guaranteed – have little incentive to work harder. Evidence from the US, Canada and Norway suggests that the volume of services provided under a salaried scheme is likely to be lower than under a fee-for-service alternative.

Supplier-induced demand – does it exist?

It is likely that the volume of services provided by clinicians will vary according to the incentives they face. However, there has been much debate within the health economics community about the existence of supplier-induced demand. Although a greater volume of services is likely to be provided under fee-for-service than under salaried schemes, this might be because lazy salaried doctors are denying patients effective care, rather than fee-for-service doctors inducing demand for unnecessary treatment. However, whereas many studies demonstrate variations in practice associated with different forms of physician remuneration, measuring the extent to which higher volumes of care represent supplier-induced demand is problematic.

Consumer moral hazard and co-payments

Another means of countering moral hazard in third-party payment systems, this time on the part of the consumer, is the use of co-payments. Many healthcare systems require patients to pay something towards the cost of investigation or treatment. This 'co-payment' might be some percentage of cost or a flat fee and, in addition to raising revenue, the aim is to limit the extent of consumer moral hazard. In other words, if the cost to patients of treatment is greater than zero, the incentive to overconsume will be reduced.

One of the problems with co-payment systems is that having to pay for care might reduce appropriate demand. The WHO has noted that 'the use of co-payments has the effect of rationing the use of a specific intervention but does not have the effect of rationalising its demand by consumers'. As the RAND health insurance experiment illustrates (Box 2.5), co-payments have important consequences for equity because it is the poor who reduce their consumption of care the most when faced with charges.

The widening resource gap between supply and demand

The increased demand for healthcare cannot be attributed entirely to moral hazard. Other factors contributing include:

- an ageing population (absolute and relative)
- technological advances
- public demand (increased awareness, expectations and mobilisation, e.g. patient advocacy groups such as the Multiple Sclerosis Society).

What can be done to manage the gap between supply and demand?

Supply-side policies. These could be pursued in an effort to increase the resources available:

- increase revenue from tax or insurance
- shift expenditure priorities (where the payer's remit is wider than health – put more government money into education perhaps)
- encourage private insurance or out-of-pocket payment
- introduce/increase charges
- increase efficiency (i.e. a better use of existing resources to enable additional activity to be undertaken from the same budget). This is of course where the tools of health economics come in.

Box 2.5 The RAND health insurance experiment – key points (Lohr et al 1986)

- The experiment took place between 1974 and 1977 at six sites in the US
- Some families had full insurance cover for healthcare costs; the rest had to pay a percentage of the cost of care. This percentage ranged from 25% to 95% but there was an upper limit on out-of-pocket expenditure
- The percentage payable by families was negatively associated with health service use, i.e. the higher the percentage paid by the consumer, the fewer services they used
- Per capita medical expenses on the free plan were 45% higher than for those who paid 95% of their expenses
- Adults who contributed to the cost of their care were significantly lower users of services than were those on the free plan
- Poorer adults used fewer services and, on some indicators, had worse outcomes than their richer counterparts
- Children from poor families were lower users of highly effective ambulatory care than their rich counterparts.

Demand-side policies. These could be pursed in an effort to reduce demands on the system:

- explicit rules about entitlement/service availability
- raising costs of access (geography, information, waiting lists, charges, etc.)
- professional autonomy to achieve pragmatic match of supply and demand.

CONCLUSIONS

What can economic theory tell us about health systems? Globally, cost containment is a high priority in healthcare systems. The gap between the demand for and supply of healthcare has prompted a reassessment of funding mechanisms within healthcare systems in many countries. Economics can explain why healthcare provision cannot be left to the vagaries of an unregulated market. More than that though, it provides some guidance on the likely consequences for equity and efficiency of alternative means of funding healthcare. It also helps explain why different groups and individuals will adopt different perspectives according to their place in the healthcare system and the incentive structures facing them. Whereas economists argue about the extent to which variations in clinical practice represent induced demand, there is clear evidence that clinician behaviour varies in response to alternative remuneration systems. This suggests that, for example, where fee-for-service schemes are in place it would make sense to target fees towards specific health goals rather than simply reward volume.

It should be remembered, however, that the goals of healthcare systems are complex and the expectations of a healthcare system will reflect the underlying value system of the country in which it is based. Healthcare systems might be as concerned to provide symbolic reassurance to the public as they are to address issues of equity and efficiency. In addition, it is worth remembering that, regardless of the economic arguments, health system reform that is designed to increase equity and/or efficiency in healthcare can fail if it is not in tune with community values or if it flies in the face of powerful interest groups (e.g. doctors, healthcare insurers) within a community.

REFERENCES

Jowell R, Curtice J, Park A et al (eds) 1998 British and European social attitudes — how Britain differs. Ashgate, Aldershot

Lohr K N, Brook R H, Kamberg C J et al 1986 Use of medical care in the RAND Health Insurance Experiment: diagnosis- and service-specific analyses in a randomized controlled trial, R-3469-HHS. RAND, Santa Monica, CA

OECD health data 2000

Ubel P A, DeKay M L, Baron J, Asch D A Cost effectiveness analysis in a setting of budget constraints — is it equitable? New England Journal of Medicine 1996; 334:1174–1177

Wanless D 2001 Securing our future health: taking a long-term view. Final report of the healthcare trends review team. HM Treasury, London

WHO 2001 The World Health Report 2000. Health systems: improving performance. WHO, Geneva. Online. Available: http://www.who.int/whr2001/2001/archives/2000/en/contents.htm

FURTHER READING

Donaldson C, Gerard K 1993 Economics of healthcare financing: the visible hand. Macmillan, Basingstoke, UK

Mossialos E, Dixon A, Figueras J, Kutzin J 2002 Funding healthcare: options for Europe. Open University Press, Buckingham, UK

Wagstaff A, van Doorslaer E 1993 Equity in health care: concepts and definitions. In: van Doorslaer E, Wagstaff A, Rutten F, eds. Equity in the finance and delivery of healthcare: an international perspective. Oxford University Press, Oxford

The economics of healthcare and healthcare systems

The public policy context for pharmacoeconomics

3

INTRODUCTION

The economic evaluation of pharmaceuticals is of growing importance and this chapter outlines the policy context in which these analyses are conducted and used. We will also highlight the tension between containing costs and promoting cost-effective technologies and examine the extent to which **pharmacoeconomics** can be of assistance to real-world decision makers.

GOVERNMENTS AND HEALTHCARE

The high profile of healthcare as a policy issue means that governments have a responsibility to ensure that the welfare of the population is safeguarded (Box 3.1).

The idea of stewardship might seem to make governments very powerful but in fact it imposes constraints on healthcare decision making at the national level because governments (or even private insurers) face multiple and, at times, competing objectives. These multiple objectives arise in part because different groups of **stakeholders** want different things: for taxpayers (who – importantly – are also voters), lower taxes are preferred to higher ones but these same taxpayers are likely, at the same time, to want the best available healthcare for themselves and their families when they experience illness; for governments, containment of costs while improving the public's health might be the main objective but they might also want, for instance, to promote a pharmaceutical industry.

Box 3.1   Governments and healthcare (WHO 2001)

'Governments should be the stewards of their national resources, maintaining and improving them for the benefit of their populations. In health, this means being ultimately responsible for the careful management of their citizens' well-being. Stewardship in health is the very essence of good government. For every country it means establishing the best and fairest health system possible. The health of the people must always be a national priority: government responsibility for it is continuous and permanent. Ministries of health must take on a large part of the stewardship of health systems.'

> **Concept box 3.1 – Rationing**
>
> Rationing in healthcare takes place when choices have to be made between beneficial healthcare technologies because the demand for the technology is greater than supply. Rationing is also known as 'priority setting' and can be undertaken explicitly or implicitly.

Governments or insurers do not have unlimited resources and are often faced with potentially huge demands for healthcare and are being asked to fund increasingly expensive medical technologies. They are therefore required to make difficult decisions about which interventions they will and will not fund, and for which patients. These decisions form the basis of **rationing** in the health service. Although patients or healthcare workers might see such rationing as inappropriate or merely as governments trying to spend less, in the context of limited resources, these decisions are an inescapable fact of life.

Pharmacoeconomics aims to inform decision makers of the relative cost effectiveness of health technologies (specifically new medicines) and might seem to provide a rational approach to rationing. However, the extent to which data on the relative cost effectiveness of medicines can be used to inform rationing decisions can be limited by the following:

- *Affordability*: if there is no money to fund a new intervention, regardless of how efficient it is, then it cannot be provided. However, a budget analysis might be performed to see if there is anything less efficient that could be dropped to free up resources.
- *Practicality*: it might be politically difficult to refuse a high profile drug even if the drug is inefficient (see Box 3.5, p 46). This is especially true if well-organised and informed patient or professional associations are involved.

Supporting the pharmaceutical industry

Many European countries have large manufacturing- and/or research-oriented pharmaceutical industries, which are often major export earners and employers. Most countries would be keen to promote their industry and would be reluctant to restrain too much activity in their home market. For example, it would be difficult for the French government to refuse to reimburse a drug developed and manufactured in France (even if it was not the most effective or efficient drug). It would also send signals to other countries – if a drug cannot achieve a market in its home country, why should any other country accept it? In addition, governments with responsibility for public health should encourage the development of new and effective drugs in areas where previously therapy has been limited. Many countries therefore have different ways of promoting their home industry.

However, this support for home industry is perhaps undermined by mergers that create huge multinational pharmaceutical companies (Box 3.2).

This redefines what constitutes a 'home market' as companies who feel they have been treated unfairly can threaten to transfer research or production to other facilities in other countries. Whereas this approach might reduce the ability of governments to control the pharmaceutical industry, it can also result in less concern for the industry. Some countries (e.g. New Zealand) have made a conscious decision to dispense with a local industry for the sake of lower drug prices. Countries that have limited home-based pharmaceutical industries (e.g. Australia and Canada) have a freer hand when it comes to cost-containment measures than the home countries of large multinational exporting companies (e.g. UK and Switzerland).

Similar issues are associated with the **drug regulation** process. Recently, thanks to harmonisation of drug regulation within Europe, this is increasingly undertaken at an international level. It is claimed that this has increased the **effectiveness** and efficiency of the drug regulation process. This is because the move away from distinctive national registration requirements has reduced the need for governments to maintain their own regulatory bureaucracy. In addition, by having a central process to cover many countries, costs are reduced for the pharmaceutical industry. What this also means, however, is that the powers of individual nation states in relation to the regulation of pharmaceuticals is diminished.

The drive for cost containment in healthcare

The rising costs of healthcare and the growing gap between supply and demand for healthcare are sources of continuing concern for **third-party payers** globally and **cost containment** in healthcare is high on the agenda of governments world wide. Reasons for increased spending on medicines and on other areas of healthcare include:

- an ageing population (absolute and relative) with increased morbidity
- technological innovation, in part extending therapy into new areas, in part displacing existing therapies
- public demand (increased awareness, expectations and mobilisation, e.g. patient groups, the Internet)
- government public health strategies (e.g. an aggressive attempt by government in the UK to reduce mortality from ischaemic heart disease has greatly increased spending on statins to lower cholesterol).

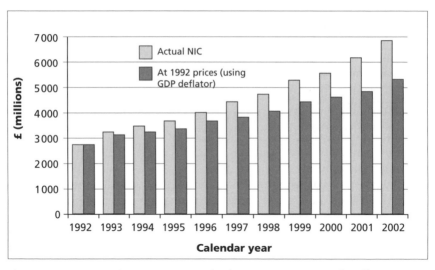

Fig 3.1 Drug costs in the community in England 1992–2002 (UK Dept of Health). NIC: net ingredient Cost; GDP: gross domestic product. DoH.

Table 3.1   Comparative drug expenditure across OECD countries, 1995 (the last year for which full data are available) (OECD 2000)

Country	Total expenditure per head (£ cash)	% GDP (public only)
Ireland	76.92	0.5
UK	87.06	0.7
Greece	88.80	1.2
Australia	90.69	0.5
Canada	102.18	0.4
Italy	105.69	0.6
Netherlands	110.02	0.6
Spain	111.17	1.1
Portugal	116.62	1.4
Denmark	120.80	0.4
Germany	155.15	1.0
Belgium	171.00	0.6
USA	197.86	0.2
France	201.25	1.0
Japan	276.70	1.0

The result is a rise in healthcare spending and medicines spending (Fig. 3.1); pharmaceutical expenditure per capita in selected OECD countries is presented in Table 3.1.

Faced with rising costs, those who pay for healthcare have been keen to contain these rises, wherever possible. Medicines are a particularly attractive area in which to try to contain costs for the following reasons:

- their costs are easily identified
- less expensive alternatives might be available (although possibly with less effectiveness)
- the major stakeholder who will be upset is neither the patient nor the healthcare professional but the pharmaceutical industry, whose complaints can often be dismissed as those of an interested party keen to boost its own profits.

In prescribing, cost containment has involved campaigns to reduce wasteful prescribing or to increase the use of generic medicines. But governments are not just keen to contain costs. They also want to use their limited resources effectively and efficiently. To achieve this, proponents of **evidence-based medicine** (EBM) argue that many medical interventions have not been evaluated and might be wasteful or even harmful to patients, and that we should practise in a way that has been scientifically proven to be effective. EBM identifies the benefits of a particular mode of treatment, usually based on the '**gold standard**' of the randomised controlled trial (RCT). The expansion of EBM means that there is an increasing volume of evidence in existence on which to conduct economic evaluations. This is especially true for pharmaceutical products. In addition, it also appears that economic evaluation, which feeds on the evidence of clinical effectiveness, might offer a scientific way to identify opportunities to improve efficiency. However, economic evaluation will often depend on less rigorous forms of evidence such as case-control studies, audit or even just expert opinion, as we shall see in later chapters.

Medicines and economic evaluation

The growth in pharmacoeconomics can be seen as part of this general concern with cost containment and efficiency but other factors can also explain why the focus of economic evaluations is primarily on pharmaceutical products rather than on other aspects of health services:

- The quality of evidence around new drug therapies is often very high – partly as a result of the rigorous requirements of **drug licensing**. This means that there are lots of data to support economic evaluations, in contrast to, for instance, most surgical procedures or other interventions.

Concept box 3.2 – Evidence-based medicine

Evidence-based medicine is an approach to healthcare practice in which clinicians have up-to-date knowledge of the evidence supporting their clinical practice, and are aware of the strength of that evidence.

- The costs of medicines have a high profile and are easily identifiable, whereas the costs of other interventions might be spread across several budgets and are therefore not so clearly identifiable. The fact that in many countries prescribing has been the fastest-growing element in the healthcare budget in recent years has also encouraged payers to investigate the costs and benefits of pharmaceutical products.
- The process for approving new drugs is very different to that in other areas. Gradual incremental service changes – an extra nurse here, some more home care there – might not be subject to rigorous scrutiny in the same way as new drugs. For drugs, specific procedures in terms of licensing and **reimbursement** make new drugs subject to specific scrutiny in a way which other types of health service development are not.
- The nature of costs incurred in the delivery of health services plays a key role in economic evaluation. If drugs are not prescribed then any reduction in total **acquisition costs** represents real savings to payers. However, if hospital admissions, for example, are prevented then these often represent only notional financial savings. Having one less patient on a ward does not permit any reduction in the major cost items such as staffing. To realise real, as opposed to notional, savings would require a ward closure. For this reason, the economic evaluation of drugs, as opposed to other services, is more attractive. Similarly, a high-cost, innovative drug will often require additional resources, rather than displacement of existing uses of resources. The issue of inadequate resources for inpatient care can be manifest in the form of waiting lists for elective patients or trolley waits for emergency care. Inadequate resources for the purchase of new drugs is likely to result in a more explicit form of rationing – an outright denial of medicine to some potential recipients. If explicit rationing of new drugs is to be undertaken then there is a need to evaluate the costs and benefits of drugs systematically to provide legitimacy for unpopular rationing decisions.
- Pharmaceutical companies are actively engaged in marketing their products in an era of cost containment. This means they might want to use economic evaluation for their products to demonstrate cost effectiveness to payers and prescribers.
- Some countries (e.g. Australia) require pharmacoeconomic submissions as part of the drug reimbursement process.

TACKLING THE RISING DRUGS BILL

Governments can pursue various initiatives to tackle the rising drug bill (e.g. **user charges**, prescriber incentives). After discussing these, we will look at measures designed to assess cost effectiveness in relation to drugs (i.e. the requirement of pharmacoeconomic data as part of the drug reimbursement process) and discuss the implications of these.

The measures that can be used in an attempt to contain rising drug costs can be broadly classified as being aimed at influencing one of the following three groups:

- prescribers
- patients
- the pharmaceutical industry.

Influencing prescribers

Here, a range of measures have been adopted, including:

- financial incentives/disincentives
- formularies and guidelines
- education and feedback to clinicians.

Financial incentives/disincentives

Various financial sticks and carrots have been used to contain drug costs. These include both schemes that reward prescribers for saving money and schemes that threaten financial penalties for overspending. The evidence suggests that financial incentives, either personal or more indirect, can have a major influence on medical practice (Box 3.3).

In the UK and in New Zealand, some GPs have been allowed to hold the budget for their prescribing and to use any savings from their prescribing budgets in other ways for the benefit of their patients. Although this resulted in short-term savings as doctors moved to generic prescribing or therapeutic substitution (i.e. using less expensive but clinically equivalent drugs), inevitably, once the one-off savings had been achieved, there was little to be gained and doctors became disenchanted with the schemes.

Although financial incentives or disincentives can produce savings, they might also adversely affect the quality of care or shift costs to other sectors of the healthcare system, such as hospital care. The morality of doctors accepting incentives to perhaps limit prescribing also needs to be considered carefully. In UK studies, doctors were willing to save money where clinically acceptable but not when it impinged on patient well-being. In the US, some states now require disclosure of any such incentives to patients, because in some cases patients were not being told of more expensive and possibly more effective alternatives to the treatments provided, at the insistence of the third-party payer.

Formularies and guidelines

Formularies are restricted lists of medicines to which prescribers are encouraged or required to adhere. The aim is to achieve consistency in prescribing

---

Box 3.3   Financial incentives in Germany

In Germany, budgetary restrictions were introduced in January 1993 that placed a ceiling on drug expenditure. The first DM280m (£90m) spent above this limit was to be paid for out of physicians' remuneration budgets. The result was that spending on drugs was 25% lower in 1993 than in 1992.

and formularies can help to contain costs by encouraging the use of generic prescribing and restricting the use of more expensive medicines. At the broadest level, formularies represent a list of medicines that are reimbursed by third-party payers, for example, many US **health maintenance organisations** (HMOs) have a defined formulary for their patients – drugs outside this might not be reimbursed. In some cases this can amount to a national reimbursement list (e.g. Australia).

Many formularies are used locally in defined areas, or even by single doctors. Limited evidence from observational studies suggests that local formularies encourage doctors to prescribe more cost effectively.

Guidelines might perhaps be seen as superior to formularies because they consider drug choice in the context of overall patient management. However, costs might not be reduced as a result of guidelines, which should be aimed at improving medical practice and which might actually increase costs. Unlike formularies, a great deal of research has gone into assessing the impact of guidelines on clinician behaviour and there is now a large body of literature determining how best to develop guidelines. When backed up with a well-constructed process of implementation, guidelines can change clinical practice and improve patient outcomes.

Education and feedback to clinicians

The best example of this is PACT (**p**rescribing **a**nalyses and **c**ost) data in the UK. This is based on all prescriptions issued by GPs and is fed back to the GPs to increase their awareness of prescribing activity and costs. Ideally, by studying this information, GPs can examine how their own practice's prescribing compares with local or national averages and be motivated to reduce variations and costs. In practice, feedback alone has little effect but it can be a vital part of an overall package of measures, including academic detailing, education and incentives, which can be very effective.

Influencing patients

Various policies have been employed to reduce demand for drugs or transfer the costs of drugs from third-party payers to consumers by asking the consumer to pay part of the cost of a medicine. Consumer charges for drugs (or co-payments) can take the form of a flat rate fee (as in the UK), a percentage fee that reflects the price of the drugs concerned (e.g. Greece) or a mixture of the two (e.g. Italy). Direct co-payments for drugs are not related to ability to pay and fall more heavily onto the less privileged groups in society. Many countries have safety nets, such as exemptions or ceilings on co-payment levels, to counter these potential negative effects.

The impact of cost sharing on patients has been the subject of a number of studies. Broadly, these indicate that increases in charges lead to a reduction in the demand for prescriptions of both effective and less effective medicines. There is therefore no guarantee that this reduced demand represents an efficiency saving (Box 3.4).

Another way to shift costs from the third-party payer onto the patient is to change the status of drugs previously classified as prescription-only medicines (POM) to over-the-counter (OTC, i.e. no prescription required). By removing the requirement for patients to contact prescribers, the policy can be sold as an expansion of consumer freedom, while at the same time it reduces both the demand on prescriber time and the pressures on drug expenditure. In practice, this seems to make little difference – one study in the UK showed that the only health-service saving from the deregulation of a range of medicines came from reduced prescription of aciclovir cream for minor cold sores. Pharmaceutical companies tend to push for such deregulation of their products as they near the end of their patent protection.

Third-party payers can also reduce demand for drugs by withdrawing reimbursement for them. This means that patients have to meet the full cost of these drugs. However, withdrawing payment for medicines does not necessarily result in savings. Studies from the US and Ireland indicate that such policies can result in an increase in drugs prescribed overall, with replacement drugs in many cases being more expensive than those previously prescribed (e.g. ranitidine for a delisted antacid).

Influencing industry

Drug reimbursement

An increasing number of governments include economic factors when deciding whether to reimburse medicines. Many governments restrict publicly reimbursed drugs by positive lists (Australia, New Zealand, Italy, France) or negative lists (Germany, Ireland, the Netherlands, Spain, UK). The former define all products that can be reimbursed, whereas the latter define all products excluded from the reimbursement process. Decisions are based on information about safety and **efficacy**, professional opinion and, in some cases, cost effectiveness.

The drug licensing process has created three hurdles that require manufacturers to demonstrate that medicines are safe, efficacious and produced under high-quality conditions. The requirement to demonstrate cost effectiveness would therefore represent a fourth hurdle for manufacturers to clear and the term 'fourth hurdle' is often used to describe this.

Australia was one of the first countries to require data on cost effectiveness before reimbursement approval. Drug manufacturers are required to submit a detailed pharmacoeconomic assessment, the content of which is carefully specified. This pharmacoeconomic submission forms the basis of subsequent price negotiations between the company and the government. The guidelines give considerable detail about the form of the economic evaluation, although companies have some leeway to argue for a specific type of analysis depending on the nature of the product. This approach has prevented the reimbursement of drugs such as beta interferon and dornase alfa in Australia, which has caused great controversy. It should be borne in mind, however, that it is in part Australia's lack of a strong, indigenous, research-oriented pharmaceutical industry that makes such action possible.

Box 3.5   The cost-effectiveness of beta interferon

The NICE-commissioned economic appraisal of beta interferon suggested that only some patients (not identifiable in advance) would respond to this expensive drug. The average cost per QALY values for all patients was well in excess of the usual NICE threshold. But if the analyses were restricted to only those patients who responded, the cost/QALY was much better. The UK Government has entered into a risk-sharing agreement with manufacturers which will entail Government funding the use of the drug in patients who are seen to respond by objective criteria but not in those who are seen not to benefit from it. Was this a realistic use of outcomes research to optimise patient benefit and resource use, or an attempt to avoid upsetting the product manufacturers and the public by engaging in explicit rationing?

Other countries have started to use pharmacoeconomic information in their deliberations on product reimbursement, although not many have gone as far as Australia. In the UK, the National Institute for Clinical Excellence (NICE) appraises the clinical cost effectiveness of selected new drugs and technologies (Box 3.5). Manufacturers whose products are selected for appraisal are required to submit pharmacoeconomic data in support of their product.

In theory, under NICE rules, if the ratio of costs to benefits is too high then reimbursement from public sector funds can be denied. However, so far this has rarely been the case: NICE has refused few health technologies and some feel that it has failed in any role of rationing.

Price controls

In many countries, governments intervene in the drug pricing process. This can take the form of **reference pricing** or the specification of more general price controls. Alternatively, attempts might be made to influence prices indirectly by setting limits to the allowable profits of drug manufacturers.

Reference pricing. This entails the establishment of a reimbursement price for a therapeutic category of drugs. Patients pay any difference between the cost of the product prescribed and the reference price. The reference price might be the average price of drugs in a category (as in the Netherlands or Germany), the lowest priced drug (as in New Zealand) or the lowest priced generic drug plus some additional amount (as in Sweden).

Profit controls. The best example of this is in the UK, where under the Pharmaceutical Price Regulation Scheme (PPRS) the pharmaceutical industry is largely free to set market launch prices as it sees fit. Instead of price controls, the approach has been to restrict profits via the PPRS. This is a voluntary agreement between the Department of Health and the Association of the British Pharmaceutical Industry (ABPI). The details of the scheme are renegotiated periodically but essentially its aim is to prevent companies from making excess profits from their sales to the NHS while at the same time recognising their need to make a reasonable return on investments, and so encourage an active pharmaceutical industry in the UK. The limits of returns are generous: 25% of capital invested, after allowing for research costs. Any profit over this can be reclaimed by the Treasury and any underachieving of target profit will allow a company a price rise in the following year. Additionally, limits are placed on marketing expenditure. Companies likely to earn excess profits can negotiate to cut drug prices, e.g. in 2000, statin prices were negotiated down in such a deal.

In France, nationally negotiated limits of sales of a drug have a similar effect.

PHARMACOECONOMICS IN PRACTICE

We now focus on pharmacoeconomic evaluation and its role in the decision-making process in practice. We will see that there are major barriers to the use of economic evaluation in practice, which go beyond methodological concerns, and we will question the extent to which relatively simple evaluations can be of use to decision makers given the complexity of the policy context in which they are operating.

The pharmaceutical industry and pharmacoeconomic evaluation

An industry view of this is presented in Chapter 4. Health service sources and health economists are commenting increasingly on the industry's use of pharmacoeconomics as it impinges on the health services (Box 3.6).

In addition to the factors described earlier in this chapter, the requirement in countries such as Australia and the UK for pharmaceutical companies to submit economic data as part of the reimbursement decision process has led to an increase in pharmacoeconomic evaluation in the pharmaceutical industry. However, leaving aside this requirement, in recent years pharmaceutical companies have become increasingly active in sponsoring or conducting economic evaluations for marketing purposes.

Although there are methodological principles to which those undertaking pharmacoeconomic evaluations are expected to adhere, there can be a tension between the desire to show favourable outcomes in terms of costs and benefits and the desire to adhere to guidelines or scientific principles in

---

Box 3.6   Pharmacoeconomics (Morgan et al 2000)

'Private corporations now finance so many aspects of health economics ... that the profession as a whole runs the risk of being co-opted ... there has been such a flurry of activity around pharmacoeconomics that outsiders often assume health economics and economic evaluation are synonymous.'

conducting analyses. The suggestion has been made on a number of occasions that these tensions might lead to bias in studies sponsored by the pharmaceutical industry.

Evidence from Australia suggests that when submitting those pharmaco-economic evaluations required for the purposes of regulation, manufacturers tend to interpret clinical data in a more favourable light than regulators. This is supported by experiences in the UK from the NICE evaluation process. In published economic evaluations, there is also evidence of a relationship between funding source and the extent to which results are favourable (Box 3.7).

The issue of bias in economic evaluation is much debated but a perception of bias in industry-funded studies is important because it can reduce their credibility in the eyes of healthcare funders. Indeed, those making decisions about drugs within health systems often consider that such studies lack credibility.

Economic evaluation and decision making in practice

Health economists have only recently begun to ask what the impact of the increased number of analyses has had on healthcare decision making. The best example of its use comes from the US, where the state of Oregon has undertaken a process of explicit priority setting for healthcare on a systematic basis rather than implicit rationing. It extended eligibility for Medicaid, a publicly funded programme of healthcare for the poor, by including in the programme all citizens with an income at or below 100% of the federally defined poverty level. To keep this affordable, it restricted the services that were provided. A process of health economic evaluation and clinical advice was used to rank possible services. The health economic approach was by **cost utility analysis** and seemed to produce many anomalies, for example that liver transplant for alcohol abuse was a better buy (in cost/**quality-adjusted life-years**; QALY) than for chronic hepatitis. Although this might be true, it was not considered acceptable to prioritise a self-inflicted problem over a problem acquired in a blameless manner. Public consultation was conducted (with some difficulty to ensure that those involved were representative of the population) to define what the delivered care packages would be.

The Oregon health plan originally included the bulk of preventive and curative services, with high priority being attached to palliative care as a result of values identified during the public consultations. The principal exclusions were the treatment of self-limiting conditions and conditions where no effective interventions were available. The basic package has expanded with time, partly because of developments in healthcare technology and partly because of new evidence that challenges earlier decisions to exclude treatments. It has also been driven by the experience of implementing the original list of services and the need to make adjustments based on advice received from clinicians. The administrators have also been reluctant to increase the restrictions in services provided, so that in Oregon explicit priority setting tended to result in inflation of a basic healthcare package.

Despite its flaws, the Oregon experience is the only case in the world where explicit priority setting has been taken so far: funding healthcare services according to priority ranking, assessing the effects of this policy and adapting it as needed each year.

Elsewhere, few governments or local authorities have embraced economic evaluations in the same way, even in pharmacoeconomics. From the small number of studies available, the suggestion is that there is, at best, only limited use of economic evaluation by decision makers at a local or national level.

One study asked health authority **prescribing advisers** (doctors and pharmacists funded to support initiatives to improve prescribing) in the UK why they did not make more use of economic evaluations. The identified barriers to the use of economic evaluation include technical issues such as inadequate information, concerns about bias, or problems relating to the extrapolation of the results of studies from one setting to another (Box 3.8).

Box 3.8   Barriers to the use of economic evaluation in prescribing (Drummond et al 1997)

- Multiple objectives are being pursued, of which efficiency is just one, and often not the most important
- It was difficult to free resources from existing services
- Industry-funded studies were seen as not credible
- Studies concerned global healthcare costs over a long period – prescribers were interested only in a limited medicines budget and could rarely see beyond the end of the financial year.

The authors conclude that NHS reforms increased the potential to use such evaluations but that there was a need to help end-users understand both them and the methodology. Major barriers to their implementation were the multiple and sometimes conflicting objectives being pursued – of which efficiency is only one – and difficulties of freeing resources from existing services to divert them to more cost-effective uses.

This might suggest that more studies and more data would increase the use of economic evaluation by decision makers. However, on closer inspection there were other barriers, which suggests that the problems might not be so readily amenable to resolution. The fact that savings identified are notional rather than real makes life difficult for those charged with balancing real, as opposed to notional, budgets. A further obstacle is that the objectives pursued in the healthcare context are often multiple and complex. For example, although citizens support the cost-effective use of resources, they are also in favour of **equity**, and the evidence suggests that they are willing to sacrifice efficiency for equity.

Barriers in a survey of prescribing advisers

Boxes 3.9, 3.10 and 3.11 discuss several of the studies that have investigated the different barriers to prescribing.

Box 3.9   The National Institute for Clinical Excellence (NICE)

NICE is a special UK NHS health authority charged with, among other activities, evaluating new and existing health technologies including medicines and making recommendations about whether they should be used in the UK NHS. NICE considers only licensed therapies and does not address issues of safety or efficacy, which are the remit of the licensing authority. The technologies to be assessed are selected by the Department of Health. The process of evaluation is two-fold. First, a technology assessment is conducted by academic units contracted to NICE and includes a review of the evidence available on a technology and an economic evaluation. Second, an appraisal or interpretation of the evidence by a NICE appraisal committee is carried out. The appraisals committee will also consider evidence presented by stakeholders (such as companies sponsoring a technology or medicine, professional or patient groups). Its judgement will be also influenced not just by the evaluations and assessments presented but also by the ethical, social and financial implications of the technology. The appraisal is published as a draft for comment before a final appraisal is issued. Stakeholders can appeal against its decisions.

NICE requests that economic evaluations should take the form of cost-utility analyses (see Chapter 7), although other methods of analysis are acceptable if appropriate. There is no fixed ceiling for the cost/QALY for a technology to be approved, although existing approvals suggest that an informal target is around £30 000 (€46 000) per QALY (Raftery 2002).

It is not the role of NICE to consider the affordability of a technology; this is the role of the Secretary of State for Health, a government minister who can accept or reject NICE advice. So far, it has always been accepted. Since 2002, local health organisations have been obliged to provide the funding for any technology approved by NICE. This raises concern about technology capture, that is, more and more NHS resources being devoted to newly evaluated technologies rather than to older, less well-evaluated but important interventions. It also causes tensions between central and local priority setting in the NHS.

It typically takes about 30 months from the time a technology is listed for review to the release of the final appraisal document and during this time many NHS organisations will not provide the health technology and patients are deprived of an effective therapy – a condition known as 'NICE blight'.

Box 3.10   Putting health economics into practice (Duthie et al 1999)

Selected GPs, health authority staff and hospital staff were interviewed to consider their potential for using health economics in practice. The broad conclusions were that health economics was of limited value because health economists did not understand NHS structures and constraints, budget setting and contracting. Hence their advice was often impractical or irrelevant. In particular, the inability to transfer funds between budgets was an important factor limiting their applicability.

Robinson (1999) considered why economic approaches to priority setting have had only limited impact in practice in the UK NHS. He argues that obstacles to the take-up of the economic approach centre on:

- limitations in the theory and practice of economic evaluations
- the nature of the wider context within which decisions on priority setting take place.

On the first point, he argues that, despite advances in research methods, there is still debate about the theoretical basis of measures typically used in economic evaluations such as the QALY, and that much of the extant empirical data is of questionable quality. In practice, this point – although also raised by other health economists – is not an issue for decision makers, perhaps reflecting their limited understanding and that they are more used to dealing with harder sciences. On the second point, Robinson maintains that politicians, healthcare professionals and local people attach importance to other factors besides allocative efficiency. This was not intended as a criticism but by way of clarification to health economists. He did not address questions about the inflexibility of NHS structures. He concluded that if economic approaches are to have more impact in the future, health economists need to adopt a wider research agenda, focusing on public-sector decision making and, in particular, on the incentives and constraints governing the use of economic data in different types of healthcare organisations, that is, less theory and more reality testing.

European studies have tended to the same conclusions: that despite goodwill towards the use of economic evaluation, few decision makers across Europe understand the methodology and hence the results are poorly applied in decision making.

A study from Canada, which examined priority-setting decisions for new cancer drugs, adds to our understanding of priority setting because it used observation of processes over time rather than surveys or interviews to capture what decision makers do. This study suggests that **cost-effectiveness analysis** was not a primary consideration in the decision process; rather, the decision-making committee approved drugs that it felt justified funding (and clinical benefit was the primary factor influencing decisions). Rather than restricting drugs to a fixed budget, the committee then requested sufficient funds to support these decisions.

Box 3.11   Guidance for manufacturers and sponsors

NICE publishes guidance for manufacturers and sponsors (e.g. patient or professional groups) on how to make submissions. This is shortly to be revised. Some key points are:

- The perspective is that of the NHS and Personal Social Service (PSS) decision maker (i.e. direct state funding)
- The clinical problem, the patient group (e.g. age and sex distribution and co-morbidities), the comparators and the treatment context (e.g. hospital, clinic, community) should be clearly defined. Estimates of patient numbers (incidence and prevalence) and recent trends in these figures should be included
- The analysis should be a cost-effectiveness analysis or cost-utility analysis, as appropriate
- The time span of the analysis should cover the period in which the main health benefits and resource use are likely. This might require extrapolation (by modelling) beyond data from controlled clinical trials
- The main comparator should be the currently most frequently used intervention
- The settings, populations and methods from which data in the original studies are drawn should be described; how the data can be generalised to the NHS should be outlined
- Discount benefits at 1.5% per annum and costs are 6% per annum. Sensitivity analyses should use 6% costs and 6% for outcomes, and 6% for costs and 0% outcomes
- Manufacturers and sponsors should provide an analysis of the likely budget impact on the NHS of the use of their technology.

At its early meetings, the committee assessed the possibility of ranking drugs according to some priority measure and then funding drugs according to ranking until the fixed budget had been allocated. This type of approach is consistent with the process of priority setting advocated by many health economists. However, adopting such an approach meant that the committee was unable to agree, and that instead each drug was assessed on its own merits. What this study illustrates is that the rationales underpinning the priority-setting process were subject to change as costs for individual treatments increased, suggesting a reluctance to ration care on grounds of cost effectiveness. A range of rationales was used, as illustrated in Box 3.12. When all options were reasonable, the decision taken was to fund a range of options and let patients decide.

Box 3.12   Rationales used in priority setting: the Cancer Care Ontario Policy Advisory Committee (Martin et al 2001)

- Benefits to patients
- Presence/absence of alternative treatments
- Total population of patients affected
- Total cost to the system
- Quality of evidence
- Access to treatment
- Pressure from physician and patient groups
- Historical precedent.

The key issues across all of these examples go beyond methodological controversy and relate to the whole structure of the health service and understanding of what the role of a health service actually is.

Policy

The existence of many conflicting aims, objectives and pressures linked to the finance, organisation and delivery of healthcare might suggest that a sensible course of action for governments would be to develop a single, unified national policy to deal with pharmaceuticals. However, in practice few countries have such a unified policy around pharmaceuticals. Australia has produced a National Medicines Policy, in which it defines four key objectives:

1. Timely access to the medicines that Australians need at a cost individuals and the community can afford.
2. Medicines meeting appropriate standards of quality, safety and efficacy.
3. Quality use of medicines.
4. Maintaining a responsible and viable medicines industry.

This policy makes explicit the need to balance health needs and affordability, while ensuring value for money for the community as whole. The need for an indigenous pharmaceutical industry is stressed, in part to promote access and also for export purposes, but there is no commitment to pay for innovation rather than simply manufacturing, reflecting perhaps that the pharmaceutical industry in Australia is far less important than in the UK. The need for partnerships between the various stakeholders is stressed although the potential for conflict is recognised, for instance, the possible trade-offs between ease of access and quality use of medicines, or between quality use (where underutilisation is identified) and cost containment.

Most countries seem to prefer to keep their options open – a single policy, although providing transparency, might constrain the government's freedom of movement in its attempts to balance industry against public health against spending.

CONCLUSION

Governments globally are concerned with cost containment in the context of healthcare. This task is made difficult by the process of globalisation, which is reducing the powers of the nation state, and the need to meet the rising expectations of an enfranchised and educated workforce. In a world characterised by scarcity, economic evaluation offers a means of increasing the extent to which healthcare resources are used efficiently. However, the policy context in which resource allocation decisions are made is complicated by the fact that decision makers pursue other objectives in addition to efficiency. In this complex environment, simple solutions – such as the allocation of resources based on the cost effectiveness of health technologies – can be difficult and, at times, undesirable.

REFERENCES

Department of Health. Prescriptions Dispensed in the Community. Statistics for 1992 to 2002: Available from http://www.doh.gov.uk/Public/sb0312/sb0312.pdf

Drummond M, Cooke J, Walley T 1997 Economic evaluation under managed competition: evidence from the UK. Social Science and Medicine 45(4):583–595

Duthie T, Trueman P, Chancellor J, Diez L 1999 Research into the use of health economics in decision making in the United Kingdom – Phase II. Is health economics 'for good or evil?' Health Policy 46:143–157

Martin D K, Pater J L, Singer P A 2001 Priority-setting decisions for new cancer drugs: a qualitative case study. Lancet 358 (9294): 1676

Morgan S, Barer M L, Evans R G 2000 Health economists meet the fourth tempter: drug dependency and scientific discourse. Health Economics 9:659–667

OECD health data 2000

Raferty J 2002 NICE: faster access to modern treatments? Analysis of guidance on health technologies. British Medical Journal 323:1300–1303

Robinson R 1999 Limits to rationality: health economics, economics and priority setting. Health Policy 49:13–26

Sacristan J A, Bolanos E, Hernandez J M et al 1997 Publication bias in health economics. Pharmacoeconomics 11(3):289–291

WHO 2001 The World Health Report 2000. Health systems: improving performance. WHO, Geneva, p 116. Online. Available: http://www.who.int/whr2001/2001/archives/2000/en/contents.htm

FURTHER READING

Bloor K, Freemantle N 1996 Lessons from international experience in controlling pharmaceutical expenditure II: influencing doctors British Medical Journal 312:1525–1527

Bloor K, Maynard A, Freemantle N 1996 Lessons from international experience in controlling pharmaceutical expenditure III: regulating industry. British Medical Journal 313:33–35

Drummond M, Brown R, Fendrick AM et al 2003 Use of pharmacoeconomics information: report of the ISPOR Task Force on use of pharmacoeconomic/health economic information in healthcare decision making. Value in Health 6:407–416

Freemantle N, Bloor K 1996 Lessons from international experience in controlling pharmaceutical expenditure. I: influencing patients. British Medical Journal 312:1469–1471

National Institute for Clinical Excellence (NICE) 2001 Guidance for manufacturers and sponsors. July 2001. Online. Available: www.nice.org.uk/pdf/technicalguidanceformanufacturersandsponsors.pdf

Sculpher M, Drummond M, O'Brien B 2001 Effectiveness, efficiency and NICE. British Medical Journal 322:943–944

Walley T, Earl-Slater A, Haycox A, Bagust A 2000 An integrated national pharmaceutical policy for the UK? British Medical Journal 321:1523–1526

Pharmacoeconomics: an industry perspective

4

INTRODUCTION

This chapter explores the issues involved in **reimbursement** in some depth and, through practical examples, helps readers to apply the information to their own situation. Although, principally, we describe the benefits of incorporating, from an early stage, reimbursement requirements into the drug development process (and outline the hazards of failing to take such action), the content of this chapter is relevant for most medical technologies. We show how reimbursement is essentially a local issue and explain why it is important for corporate and local staff to work closely to improve the development process and enhance reimbursement prospects for their product. We also outline steps that pharmaceutical companies must take at each stage in the drug development process, from Phase II or earlier through to post-launch (see Concept box 8.2, p. 129 for details of phases of drug development).

REIMBURSEMENT

Ensuring reimbursement and funding for a **medical technology** is an accepted and integral step in the market access and uptake of a new medical technology (see Concept box 4.1). A development programme is incomplete if it addresses

---

Concept box 4.1 – Reimbursement

In this chapter we use the term 'reimbursement' to refer to the processes by which third-party payers – including governments, sickness funds, local authorities and managed-care organisations (MCOs) decide which drugs and medical technologies are suitable for funding. Processes include price setting, inclusion in positive lists and formularies, and clinical guidelines from organizations such as the National Institute for Clinical Excellence (NICE) in England and Wales. For convenience, this report refers to all these different processes as 'reimbursement'.

---

regulatory submission but not these crucial issues, which should be considered explicitly and systematically before substantial resources are devoted to the development process. The cost of systematic assessment at an early stage is modest and marginal compared with overall expenditure on a development programme, and analytical tools exist to perform such assessment.

Reimbursement and funding are local issues and information requirements vary between major markets and among payers. As reimbursement regulations change frequently, input from local experts should be sought. This input is most valuable before a company has committed (in Phase III) to pivotal data collection and market positioning of a medical technology. Protecting reimbursement and maintaining commitment to funding once a product has been launched is increasingly important. Companies should possess a mechanism to address these issues through Phase IV and outcomes studies.

To maximise the likelihood of successful reimbursement, a company should implement processes that meet the following objectives:

- systematic assessment of the reimbursement potential of candidate products at an early stage of development
- continuous reimbursement planning during development
- collection and utilisation of information requirements for reimbursement in key markets before the Phase III programme is finalised
- initiating and managing studies to maintain reimbursement after the launch of the medical techology, at either the affiliate or the corporate level.

Global healthcare spending

Overall spending on healthcare in the seven largest pharmaceutical markets (the US, France, Germany, Italy, Spain, the UK and Japan) has increased steadily from an average of 5.7% of **gross domestic product** in 1970 to 7.2% in 1980, 7.9% in 1990, and 9.1% in 2000 (Fig. 4.1). Healthcare payers in all the major pharmaceutical markets have tried to restrain what might appear to be an inexorable rise in expenditures by using measures such as drug price and profit controls, restrictive formularies, positive and negative lists (i.e. lists of drugs that might or might not be prescribed and reimbursed), and restrictions on reimbursed indications.

Figure 4.2 shows the use of some of these cost-containment measures in the six major European pharmaceutical markets.

Securing reimbursement does not automatically follow marketing authorisation in some major European markets. With a few exceptions, reimbursement requires separate negotiation with a national body. In some countries, for example the UK, where formal reimbursement does not exist but where multiple formal and informal bodies are key to the funding and uptake process (e.g. NICE, primary care trust (PCT) formulary committees) the picture can seem very confusing. In these cases, undertaking a review and analysis of the key information needs of the different **stakeholders**, and the most efficient way of presenting the crucial information in support of the product, is a critical part of the market access process. Failure to obtain

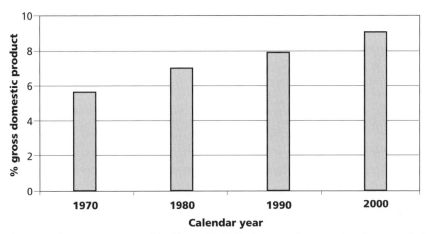

Fig 4.1 The increasing costs of healthcare (% GDP). Average of seven major pharmaceutical markets

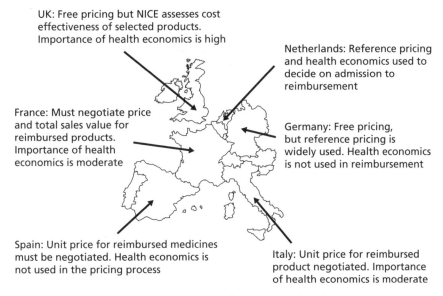

UK: Free pricing but NICE assesses cost effectiveness of selected products. Importance of health economics is high

Netherlands: Reference pricing and health economics used to decide on admission to reimbursement

France: Must negotiate price and total sales value for reimbursed products. Importance of health economics is moderate

Germany: Free pricing, but reference pricing is widely used. Health economics is not used in reimbursement

Spain: Unit price for reimbursed medicines must be negotiated. Health economics is not used in the pricing process

Italy: Unit price for reimbursed product negotiated. Importance of health economics is moderate

Fig 4.2 Restrictions to reimbursement and market access in selected European countries

reimbursement for a drug can reduce its sales substantially, although in some countries (e.g. Italy) this does not preclude sales potential. However, many pharmaceutical companies still focus their drug development programmes on marketing authorisation rather than reimbursement.

The differences between reimbursement and drug registration

The information requirements for obtaining reimbursement differ substantially from those for drug registration. The primary objective of studies for drug registration is to demonstrate the efficacy and safety of an agent. The high cost of developing drugs means that companies are under pressure to achieve a return on this investment – and in particular to file for registration – as quickly as possible. To save both time and money, drug registration studies typically have the following characteristics:

- they are placebo controlled (no active comparator if ethical) to achieve statistical significance with the smallest number of patients
- they use surrogate markers to reduce sample size and study duration
- they use restrictive entry criteria to minimise unwanted variation between patients and thus to limit the required sample size.

Such characteristics do not necessarily lend themselves to the requirements of a reimbursement submission, which has to demonstrate – usually to a body that funds healthcare – that the benefits of reimbursing a drug are sufficient to justify the cost. Reimbursement authorities seek information that allows them to:

- compare the new therapy with normal practice (which varies from setting to setting)
- evaluate the likely benefit of the new therapy to patients
- understand the impact of the new therapy on the whole group of patients in which it is likely to be used in practice
- assess the impact of the new therapy on budgets and spending.

THE IMPORTANCE OF MEETING LOCAL-COUNTRY INFORMATION REQUIREMENTS

Reimbursement is a local issue and authorities seek to understand the benefits of a new product for their own patients and the cost to their own budget (Box 4.1).

Failure to meet local information requirements can cost company revenue in three main ways:

- *Limited access to patients*: a drug for which evidence of clear superiority over existing therapies is lacking can be reimbursed in only a limited group of patients or limited to use as a second-line therapy in patients who have failed other treatments.
- *Lower price*: reimbursement bodies are interested in the benefits that a drug offers to their patients. Companies that fail to demonstrate such patient benefits are missing an opportunity to demonstrate added value to their customers and thus to command a premium price.
- *Lost time*: if a company and a reimbursement authority cannot agree on a commercially viable combination of price and reimbursed indication, the company will lose out on potential sales while it is collecting additional data to satisfy the reimbursement body.

Reimbursement bodies tend to look particularly critically at submissions for 'lifestyle drugs', 'me-too' products, line extensions and new formulations, on the grounds that such products add only limited value. It seems that they are

Box 4.1   Zanamivir – a case study on the importance of meeting local information requirements (NICE 1999)

Zanamivir, which was marketed as Relenza™ by Glaxo Wellcome (this company has since merged with SmithKline Beecham and is now called GlaxoSmithKline), received marketing approval in the UK in June 1999 for the 'treatment of ... adults and adolescents (12 years) who present with symptoms typical of influenza when influenza is circulating in the community'.

Although zanamivir was the first approved treatment for influenza (a disease that kills thousands in Europe every year), payers were initially unenthusiastic about it. In England and Wales, the National Institute for Clinical Excellence (NICE) issued guidance in October 1999 advising health professionals not to prescribe the drug during the 1999/2000 influenza season. NICE noted that '... due to the limited numbers of "high-risk" patients ... that have been treated with zanamivir in clinical trials, the Institute has not found it possible to conclude that the product reduces the frequency of serious secondary complications in these groups of patients.' Glaxo Wellcome had failed to identify the patient population that was of interest to NICE.

The company responded to this setback by conducting additional studies to demonstrate drug benefits in the relevant patient group. A second assessment by NICE, towards the end of 2000, reached a different conclusion: 'For otherwise healthy adults with influenza, the use of zanamivir is not recommended. Zanamivir is recommended, when influenza is circulating in the community, for the treatment of at-risk adults ... At-risk adults are individuals falling into one or more of the following categories: age 65 years or over; chronic respiratory disease; significant cardiovascular disease; immunocompromised; diabetes mellitus.' A third assessment is ongoing at the time of writing (November 2002).

Note that zanamivir is still not recommended for otherwise healthy adults – the main population studied in the drug development programme and described in the product license. The company lost a full year's sales and incurred the expense of additional analyses and studies because it had not generated evidence of outcomes in the correct population in Phase III.

also reluctant to authorise reimbursement for drugs that have the following characteristics:

- high potential budget impact
- high absolute price (per patient)
- high price relative to comparators
- modest outcomes benefits compared with existing therapy
- poor evidence of outcomes benefits.

To avoid rejection on these grounds, companies must systematically address reimbursement issues during development – a development programme that addresses regulatory submission data but not reimbursement data is not a complete programme.

Companies should seek to develop drugs that can demonstrate sufficient benefit to patients to justify the cost to the customer. The reimbursement submission needs to:

- provide reimbursement bodies with the information they need
- identify the patients who will benefit from the drug
- fully demonstrate the clinical, economic and patient benefits of using the drug
- be generated at reasonable cost and in a timely manner.

We will now address these issues through the classic drug development phases. This structure is one of convenience and simplicity and not intended to exclude other health technologies – the information applies just as much to these technologies, whose reimbursement processes are changing to become more in line with those used for drugs, despite differences in the research, development and registration processes.

HEALTH ECONOMICS IN EARLY DEVELOPMENT: PHASE II AND EARLIER

By the time a drug reaches Phase II testing, its developer should have assessed the reimbursement prospects of both the agent and its proposed indications. Choices relating to positioning, patient population and the evidence to be collected all influence the eventual price of a drug and the patient groups for which it is reimbursed.

Companies should consider the reimbursement potential of new compounds systematically and explicitly before devoting substantial resources to the development process. A useful analytical tool available to assist in this process is economic modelling. These analyses include the outcomes and economic characteristics of a product undertaken at an early stage of development and reveal a great deal of useful information. Early-stage models are of value to companies for several reasons:

- An early understanding of the likely reimbursement case that can be made for a target product profile informs go/no-go decisions and helps in the selection of patients and end-points.
- Structured consideration of the reimbursement potential of a product identifies key unknown details relating to the potential reimbursed price and patient numbers.
- Building a model forces firms to be explicit and quantify the assumptions that they have made about the profile of a product and the data that will be collected in studies.
- A model allows companies to interpret the impact of new data on the reimbursement potential of a product quickly and transparently.
- Reviewing reimbursement requirements and commercial objectives can and should inform data collection and study design.

Early modelling of reimbursement potential involves four stages:

1. *Modelling the management of the disease.* The first step is to produce a decision-analytical model describing the management/progress of the disease in question. Such a model describes the flow of patients through the treatment process and includes the principal treatments and outcomes (including adverse events) that influence the perceived value of the product in development to the particular reimbursement authorities. Early-stage **disease management** models are often very simple. These models need to be forward-looking. At this early stage of development, forecasting the competitive situation at time of launch is often complicated by uncertainties

surrounding other compounds in development and potential changes to treatment practice. Although it is impossible to predict these factors precisely, it is important to describe the likely management process at the time of launch as accurately and explicitly as possible in order to plan for all eventualities.

2. Modelling the costs and benefits of the new product. The next step is to define a target profile (i.e. a summary of the key attributes and market positioning of the drug) for inclusion in the previously described disease model. The target profile describes the likely costs and patient benefits of including the drug under development in the management process; it also compares these costs and patient benefits with those of the current and projected standard therapy. A refinement at this stage is to consider the development plan for the product, and thus what information will be available to reimbursement authorities at the time of launch. This exercise enables a company to determine whether the data available are strong enough to meet the reimbursement authority's standards of proof.

3. Estimating the likely maximum reimbursed price. Most reimbursement authorities have clear procedures for reimbursement application, although the transparency of their own decision-making processes does vary considerably. It is generally possible to use past decisions to estimate the criteria that the reimbursement authority applies in decision making. This information can help when estimating the likely maximum reimbursed price of a product. By combining this information with baseline epidemiological and disease-progression data, companies can estimate the number of patients available at each stage of the management model and the number of patients in any relevant subgroups. Weighing the likely benefits and cost of a new product against the reimbursement authority's presumed criteria allows a company to estimate the maximum reimbursed price for a product and the volume of available sales for the product in that indication and patient group (Box 4.2).

4. 'What if ...?' analysis. The final element of early-stage modelling is **sensitivity analysis** (a 'what if ...?' analysis). Creating a model requires quantification of the assumptions used, often on the basis of strategic documents or expert opinions. It is particularly useful to vary the assumptions and examine the resulting changes in the costs and patient benefits of using the product. Some sample questions are:

- What happens to the reimbursed price if demonstrated efficacy differs from the target profile?
- What happens to the reimbursed price and market size if a different patient group is assessed?
- What happens if the expected comparator is different or if the price of comparators is lower (or higher) than expected?

Systematic assessment can identify the key sources of uncertainty surrounding the maximum reimbursed price and potential market volume. This exercise can show a company what further information is required and what data collection is needed to improve the accuracy of the initial estimates.

Box 4.2 Using maximum reimbursed price calculations to refine the drug development process

Figure 4.3 shows an example of output from an early-stage decision model. In this case, the mechanism of action of the potential product meant that it could plausibly be developed for use in a number of different patient groups. Using the target profile for the product, the expected price of competitors and information about the costs and effectiveness of other therapies, we were able to construct a simple cost-effectiveness model of the potential product for each patient group.

We used the model to estimate the cost effectiveness of the potential product at the company's target price. We then calculated the highest price at which the product would appear to be cost effective – the maximum reimbursed price – for each patient group. The analysis showed that for three patient groups the price was relatively attractive between $1.05 and $1.50 per day, but for the fourth group the maximum reimbursed price was lower: less than $0.50 per day.

However, we then combined the findings with epidemiology data. Because of a larger number of potential patients and longer duration of treatment for each patient, the potential market size for group 4 was found to be much bigger than for the other groups.

Further analysis allowed us to show how the maximum reimbursed price varies if a different efficacy profile is used, and what would be the main risks if the price of competitors changed, or if new agents entered the market. The company was able to refine its development goals with a better estimate of the price that could be achieved in each potential patient group.

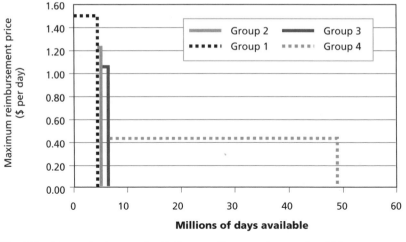

Fig 4.3 Price and volume trade-off: Germany. Base case 'expected profile'

The key contributors

The level of investment in reimbursement planning in the early stages of development should be commensurate with the probability of successful development. New chemical entities (NCEs) have a high rate of failure during development but the cost of systematic assessment at an early stage is modest compared with overall expenditure on a development programme. As the cost to a company of a product that fails to clear reimbursement after the expense of an entire development programme is extremely high, we advocate systematic consideration of reimbursement potential before a company commits substantial resources to the development of a product.

In early-stage development, the only staff with the scientific and technical knowledge to assess the likely reimbursement potential of a new product are often based in corporate functions, such as strategic marketing or clinical development. However, reimbursement is a local issue. If suitably qualified local staff are not available at this stage of development, there is a danger that the company will develop a model that describes a small number of key markets (e.g. the US and one or two major European countries) and assume that these settings will be broadly representative of the global market.

HEALTH ECONOMICS IN LATE PHASE II/PRE-PHASE III

Reimbursement decisions are made when a product is launched. The data collected and patients included in Phase III testing determine the licensed indication of the drug and hence the scope of reimbursement negotiations. It is therefore important to plan carefully in advance to ensure that Phase III studies collect data appropriate for the desired reimbursement population.

Key activities

Phase II studies

These are of limited use in generating data of value to the reimbursement process. Such studies tend to be conducted in tightly defined patient groups, involve small numbers and include close monitoring of safety. However, Phase II offers a convenient opportunity to collect baseline data on, for example, resource use and health-related quality of life (HRQoL) in a patient population. It is also possible to pilot resource use and HRQoL data collection in patients at this stage.

Phase III planning

This is a key decision point: companies often simply repeat the methodologies of their Phase II protocols and ignore useful additional information in their haste to assemble a registration package. However, Phase III planning is the last chance for input from the key markets on core data collection, and the best opportunity for companies to review study designs and assess the potential of studies to collect data to support reimbursement. Several steps need to be taken before Phase III begins. Key activities can occur in parallel with clinical studies and are as follows:

1. *Review the epidemiology of the disease.* Such reviews are intended to identify patient groups available for treatment and appropriate surrogate markers for use in pivotal studies. Reimbursement authorities generally favour information on the impact of a new drug on patient outcomes. However, to save time and money, regulatory studies tend to be powered to

63

Table 4.1 Examples of surrogate end-points and clinical outcomes

Indication	Surrogate end-point	Outcome
Coronary heart disease	Blood cholesterol	Survival
Diabetes	Blood sugar measures	Blindness, survival
HIV	CD4 cell count, viral load	Aids, quality of life, survival
Psoriasis	PASI score	Quality of life, time in remission
Infertility/IVF	Oocytes created	Live birth

show a difference in surrogate markers rather than final outcomes. One solution is to model the link between surrogate markers and final outcomes. To be suitable for modelling, a surrogate marker must be linked to a final outcome by high-quality data from a previous observational, epidemiological or experimental study. Table 4.1 provides examples of surrogate end-points and clinical outcomes.

2. Review the economic burden of the disease. Such review is multipurpose:

- To increase the political profile of a disease by demonstrating associated mortality, morbidity and economic burden.
- To quantify the main components of the cost of disease and thus identify potential cost savings from improved management of the disease.
- To assess the quality of the available economic information and whether it will be necessary to generate new (non-experimental) economic data to demonstrate the value of the product.
- To assess the quality and quantity of available data on morbidity and the impact of the disease on final patient outcomes that will be of interest to reimbursement authorities.

3. Identify comparators that are relevant to the local country. Comparators for reimbursement assessment are determined at the national level. In some cases, a particular therapy is the obvious (or even the only) suitable comparator in all markets, but national differences in treatment practice or reimbursement restrictions often necessitate multiple comparisons. For example, the existing use of oral agents in the management of type 2 diabetes varies significantly between countries, making comparisons of the newer agents, such as the glitazones, quite complex. Authorities might wish to see a new product compared with agents used commonly in local practice – acarbose in Germany, fixed combination metformin/sulfonylurea products in Italy and sulfonylureas alone in France. The relevance of all of these comparisons would be lower in the US, where proportionately more patients are managed with insulin. Companies need to identify the comparators that will be required before they commit to pivotal data collection.

4. Identify data requirements for reimbursement. Despite the existence of some common features, data requirements for reimbursement vary between countries – and sometimes even between payers within a country. An understanding of the local political situation, as well as of formal regulations, is valuable in interpreting the practical operation of reimbursement, especially in Europe. Continuing healthcare reforms mean that national requirements change frequently. Expert local knowledge (obtained from qualified staff working in the country in question) is therefore important to ensure that the company has realistically addressed the likely outcomes of reimbursement requirements in each market.

Collecting outcomes data

A key decision is whether to collect outcomes data by modifying pivotal trials or by setting up separate reimbursement-oriented studies. Data collection to support reimbursement is often 'piggybacked' onto regulatory (especially Phase III) studies for reasons of convenience, cost and speed. This is discussed further in Chapter 8. However, adding reimbursement or outcomes data to pivotal studies can have several drawbacks. It can:

- inflate the cost of the regulatory study
- delay regulatory submission by extending the study
- compromise quality
- generate information that will not help reimbursement because the comparator or patients considered might be inappropriate.

In some instances, pivotal trials are not a suitable means for collecting reimbursement data. For example, piggybacking might be too costly or time-consuming if:

- there are substantial differences between the 'gold-standard' practice required in trials and normal clinical practice
- national differences in data requirements necessitate a large number of comparators
- the targeted disease has a very long duration
- registration can be granted on an accepted surrogate marker.

In these circumstances, separate outcomes studies to support reimbursement will be more advantageous than piggybacking. Separate studies can require large numbers of patients but the additional cost is justified if they substantially improve the reimbursement prospects of the drug. Companies must choose between creating additional data to support reimbursement through new studies, modifying existing trials or using models to estimate the link between surrogate markers and outcomes. This decision should take into account the expected benefit to the company of generating better data to support reimbursement, the cost of lost sales if the reimbursed launch is delayed (either by the need for additional studies or by extended reimbursement negotiations) and the cost of additional data collection.

Clinical, commercial and outcomes research/health economics staff should participate in these activities to ensure that they support the data-collection strategy and that appropriate outcomes data are collected to the same standard as the clinical end-points.

Health economics in Phase III

Phase III clinical trials can be a very valuable source of reimbursement data. However, other, parallel actions are needed to provide robust evidence of a drug's economic and humanistic value in support of reimbursement and other market access initiatives. Economic and HRQoL data collection should be subject to the same rigorous data quality procedures as the traditional clinical efficacy and safety parameters.

This chapter does not explore the process of data collection in detail. We aim instead to describe a number of key principles that should maximise the quality and relevance of the data.

Collection of resource-use and quality-of-life data within the Phase III clinical trial programme. Companies must consider carefully the appropriateness of each trial design as a vehicle for collecting economic and HRQoL data. For example, does the trial reflect current therapeutic practice and include relevant comparator treatments? Will the results be generalisable to the target patient population or relevant only to a highly defined and controlled trial population? Given that clinical trial sample size calculations are based on the predicted treatment effect of the primary clinical end-point, is the study population sufficiently large to detect possible differences in resource use patterns or HRQoL scores (bearing in mind that variances for these kinds of data tend to be fairly large)? Will the process of additional data collection overburden either the investigators or patients?

If, on the basis of these criteria, a study is deemed appropriate for the collection of economic data, the company must then decide which items to measure. The management of many medical conditions is complex and demands numerous resources. It can be helpful to keep in mind the 80:20 rule, that is, 80% of the costs are incurred by 20% of the resource use items. Identifying and measuring only the key cost-drivers in the management process will minimise the burden of data collection.

Many studies fail to deliver robust economic or HRQoL data largely because clinical teams within the sponsor company (and the investigators themselves) do not fully support the additional data collection. They are often not involved in the process of deciding which additional data to collect, or given an explanation as to why these additional data are important to the successful commercialisation of the product. In such cases, the additional data collection is simply seen as an extra burden to already busy people. It is therefore vital to fully integrate the economic and HRQoL data collection activities into the clinical trial process. Further, both the clinical teams and investigators need to understand the reasons for the additional data collection.

Activities conducted in parallel with Phase III clinical trials. 'Bridging information' is often needed to fill the gaps between the data collected in the Phase III clinical programme and what is required to perform appropriate economic analyses. The nature and extent of these data will depend on what is being collected in the Phase III trials themselves, and on any data gaps that were identified previously in early modelling activities. Examples of the types of information that can be collected at this stage are: unit costs for resource use items and **utility** estimates to be applied in **cost utility analysis** (cost per quality-adjusted life-year [QALY] estimates).

A company might decide at this point to develop and refine **economic models** that extrapolate from surrogate end-points to **effectiveness** and cost effectiveness measures to ensure that these models are available as soon as clinical trial efficacy data are analysed. The collection of epidemiological and cost-of-illness data, used in economic evaluations and for general market support, can also be completed at this point.

Planning for further studies. The value of Phase III pivotal trials in making clinical and cost effectiveness judgements is limited because the highly selective populations and specialist academic settings of these studies are not representative of the market conditions in which the drug will eventually be used in the real-world setting. Companies should therefore consider the feasibility of conducting more naturalistic studies of the clinical, HRQoL and economic outcomes of a therapy. Such 'outcomes' studies:

- include a broad patient population with as few inclusion and exclusion criteria as possible
- compare the new therapy with current clinical practice
- are conducted in the treatment settings in which the new agent will be used in day-to-day practice
- do not introduce protocol-specific procedures, interventions, or visits.

The aim is to conform as closely as possible to 'real life' treatment patterns, thereby permitting an evaluation of the true impact of a new therapy.

Planning for reimbursement requires a series of interlinked actions during the whole development process. Input from clinical research, commercial, pricing and outcomes research/health economics staff is needed during the development process to manage planning for reimbursement.

To provide clear leadership in this process, it is helpful to establish a 'reimbursement team' in parallel with commercial and clinical development teams. This team should be charged with successful commercialisation of a product – in particular, with ensuring the reimbursed launch – rather than ensuring regulatory submission or approval.

Local markets should also be involved to refine the product positioning and update data requirements.

Planning for regulatory submission and reimbursement

Although reimbursement is a local issue, much of the product expertise required for reimbursement negotiations resides in a company's central/corporate functions. The challenge is to transfer knowledge – including valuable information on successes and failures in other countries – efficiently from head office to local affiliates. Head office also needs to coordinate local activities effectively.

The tendency to disperse development teams as soon as Phase III trials are completed can limit the expertise that is accessible to foreign affiliates when they are negotiating reimbursement (often 1–2 years after the Phase III studies have reported). This situation is an inefficient use of expensively acquired experience, knowledge, and data.

Many companies have processes for transferring study results to marketing affiliates and maintaining knowledge (e.g. by producing a product monograph or maintaining departments responsible for Phase IV studies and scientific communications). Similar arrangements should be made for the transfer of information to support the reimbursement process. A 'reimbursement dossier' for use by affiliate organisations might contain the following information:

- a summary of evidence of the epidemiology and burden of disease
- information about the impact of the product on patient outcomes and quality of life
- cost effectiveness data
- information on the likely impact of the product on customer budgets and healthcare service delivery.

Unlike the efficacy and safety of a drug, cost effectiveness, epidemiology and budget impact depend on local circumstances. Evaluations of the population, prices and funding arrangements must be customised to the requirements of an individual reimbursement agency or payer. A reimbursement dossier that fails to address these differences will not be useful to local staff members, who need a dossier supported by appropriate tools that can customise results. These tools might include epidemiological and economic models, and standard methodologies to elicit local population and observational information.

It is inefficient to repeat the process of generating a full reimbursement dossier in each separate market. Headquarters staff can coordinate the activities of local affiliates, leading to resource savings and capitalising on valuable knowledge. Such assistance should include statistical support and outcomes research/health economist support, as well as scientific expertise.

HEALTH ECONOMICS POST-LAUNCH

Reimbursement is often seen as a 'hurdle' to be cleared to gain access to the market. However, it is increasingly apparent that 'once-only' reimbursement negotiations do not adequately meet customers' needs. Reimbursement is typically based on the limited dataset – derived largely from tightly controlled clinical studies – that is available when a drug is first launched. However, data gathered from everyday practice, in a much larger population and without strict controls, might yield very different effectiveness results. In addition, the emergence of new competitors could alter the use and value of an established product.

Therefore, some markets (e.g. France and Italy) require periodic reapplication for reimbursement as new information becomes available. In England and Wales, NICE appraisals are explicitly time limited and are repeated periodically. Reassessment of reimbursement – based on new evidence on a therapy or on a comparison with new competitors – is likely to become more common in the future.

Outcomes studies in Phase IV can be used to confirm claims made at initial reimbursement and to support attempts to maintain and extend reimbursed indications and patient groups. Such studies can also raise barriers to entry for competitors if incumbents are able to demonstrate outcomes benefits that are difficult (or even impossible) to detect in regulatory studies.

Most companies have mechanisms in place for conducting Phase IV studies that have application beyond a particular country or setting. Headquarters and local staff need to work together closely to ensure that these studies are able to meet continuing reimbursement requirements.

Implications for the medical technology industry

Organisation

To minimise problems in the reimbursement process, a company needs to implement processes that meet the objectives outlined below.

Table 4.2 Key objectives and activities at each stage in the drug development process

Stage in life cycle	What to do?	Why do it?
Early development	Assess reimbursement potential of products and indications. Early modelling. Determine 'economically justifiable price' for the profile and patient group	Input to feasibility of commercialisation and to achieve a required return on investment
Before Phase III	Identify and establish minimum evidence requirements for successful reimbursement. Solicit input from local experts in key markets	Collect appropriate data in pivotal studies. Ensure data is appropriate for key markets
Phase III	Hypothesis testing in pivotal studies. Collection of supportive data in parallel to clinical studies	Main opportunity to generate core data for reimbursement
Phase IIIB	Outcomes studies. Burden of disease studies	Generate additional data on effectiveness to support efficacy
Market access	Generate 'reimbursement dossier'. Maintain sufficient central support/staffing for product during roll-out of data	Ensure effective application of core data to local markets. Prevent expensive and wasteful duplication of effort
Phase IV	Outcomes/ effectiveness studies	To maintain reimbursement. To support sales messages and formulary access

Table 4.2 provides a checklist of key objectives and activities at each stage in the drug development process.

Resources

Incorporating extra information requirements adds to the already costly drug and medical technology development process – outcomes studies can be particularly large and expensive. However, the cost of establishing reimbursement planning, associated processes and data collection should be compared with the potential cost of failing to take such action. A product that is denied reimbursement wastes many millions of dollars of research expenditure.

Companies should consider the following changes in resource allocation to incorporate reimbursement requirements more effectively into the drug development process:

- Expenditure in early development to allow early-stage assessment of reimbursement potential. This investment should result in fewer products that fail at reimbursement and improved reimbursement terms for those that succeed.
- Earlier investment by local marketing companies in planning for new products will enhance the design of Phase III studies. This need is greatest for novel drugs and for disease areas that are unfamiliar to the company.
- Making resources available in the central organisation to support the design and execution of local reimbursement strategies. This change might require that staff who would otherwise be involved in regulatory studies be allocated to supporting reimbursement.

REFERENCES

National Institute for Clinical Excellence (NICE) 1999 Guidance on the use of zanamivir (Relenza) in the treatment of influenza. NICE, London

Disease management and the technique of programme budgeting and marginal analysis

5

INTRODUCTION

This chapter explains the concept of **disease management** and examines the rationale for the trend in health services and pharmaceutical industries towards the disease management approach.

The first part of the chapter ('What is meant by disease management?') explains what is meant by the term 'disease management' and describes how this approach to patient care seeks to coordinate resources across the health-care delivery system. It illustrates how the growing interest in **evidence-based medicine**, a commitment to integrated care and the need for **cost containment** contribute to making disease management an attractive idea.

The next part ('Implementing disease management', p. 76) discusses implementation in relation to disease management. It then goes on to describe the involvement of the pharmaceutical industry in disease management initiatives within the NHS and in the US, citing examples of contributions to the delivery of healthcare. In both cases the role of **health economics** and the different approaches to assessing costs and benefits of care are outlined.

The next part ('Programme budgeting and marginal analysis', p. 78) provides an introduction to the health economic technique of **programme budgeting and marginal analysis** (PBMA) in relation to disease management and resource allocation.

The final part ('Future directions and conclusions', p. 82) examines the likely future contribution of health economics within a disease management framework.

WHAT IS DISEASE MANAGEMENT?

Background

Disease management is a term with many meanings. It can be used at a general level to simply mean managing the care of a particular condition. Alternatively, it describes a process used by the pharmaceutical industry to market its products. This is particularly prevalent in the US, where disease management programmes are used as a mechanism to negotiate with **third-party payers** (usually **health maintenance organisations**; HMOs) to contain drug costs. Others use the term to denote the development of systems and processes aimed at coordinating care to improve quality and outcomes, which might have little or no connection with the marketing activities of pharmaceutical companies.

Here, we use the term 'disease management' to refer to an approach that moves away from viewing care as a series of discrete episodes or points of contact with different parts of the healthcare system, and instead sees patients as entities experiencing the clinical course of a disease. The emphasis is on the elimination of fragmented care and its replacement by the coordination of care and resources across the healthcare system, with all costs planned and accounted for. In short, disease management aims to provide systematic, integrated, evidence-based care to patients with chronic diseases and to move away from the previous focus on individual episodes of care.

The emphasis of disease management is to get the whole system of care right, with the focus on the patient, and this approach tries to overcome problems associated with the compartmentalisation of care into discrete, uncoordinated episodes of care, reactive rather than preventive medicine and poor patient management. In addition, advocates argue that the monitoring and auditing processes of disease management approaches help assure appropriateness and thus help contain drug costs.

Disease management programmes take many forms. The variations in form and content reflect the local context in terms of the values and mechanisms underpinning the provision of healthcare in different countries. The fragmented healthcare system in the US contrasts markedly with the system in UK, for example, in which healthcare is seen as a right of citizenship, with the financing and delivery of healthcare the responsibility of the public sector. In addition, the development of disease management has been influenced by a number of very different factors (e.g. cost containment, quality improvement, reducing variations in care), which will also influence the nature of the resulting disease management approaches.

What is the rationale for the disease management approach?

Globally, third-party payers for healthcare struggle to contain costs within available resources. As with so many initiatives in healthcare management, cost containment is a major driving force for disease management. The surge in disease management approaches in the 1990s has been seen as having its origins in the activities of the pharmaceutical industry in the US. In the 1980s, cost containment in health in the US was pursued by the use of health maintenance organisations (HMOs), which aimed to reduce hospital admissions and squeeze provider **reimbursement** to save money. Standard protocols, which guided clinicians in the treatment of disease, were intended to reduce discretion and variation in care, reducing costs at the same time. Disease management in the US was a response to growing fears in the pharmaceutical industry that, with costs still rising, the HMOs would now turn their cost-cutting efforts to drug expenditure. With pharmaceutical companies having to persuade HMOs to offer their products rather than approach physicians directly, disease management programmes offered a means of gaining a place on the HMO formulary by providing an added value service. Once a company's drug was included on a formulary, the doctors were obliged – either by the patient's insurance plan or by HMO directive – to use that drug. This is in marked contrast to the UK, where GPs have the clinical freedom to prescribe their drug of choice enshrined in law.

Pharmaceutical companies were able to use their databases of information on drugs dispensed to identify those patients with chronic diseases and to offer educational services to those patients. This is a further contrast with the UK, where there are currently no uniformly available databases in primary care to identify patients in this way, and current legislation forbids identification of patients for direct targeting by pharmaceutical companies. In the US, drug companies entered into agreements with HMOs that involved redesigning care to move away from fragmentation to a disease management approach, which usually incorporated the products of the pharmaceutical company concerned.

By 1999, around 200 companies were offering disease management programmes. These programmes come in all shapes and sizes, and not all are offered by pharmaceutical companies or their offshoots. Typically, disease management packages will focus on care for chronically ill patients. In areas such as asthma and diabetes, fragmented care can result in inadequate monitoring and regulation of therapy, which in turn can precipitate an acute admission. Disease management, the theory goes, will replace fragmentation with integration and at the same time reduce costs. Such schemes have helped reduce cost escalation to 'European' levels, at least temporarily (Anderson 1997, Fagan 1998)

Faced with a desire from third-party payers to contain costs, pharmaceutical companies used disease management approaches to illustrate the cost of drug therapy in the context of the total cost of the disease. By quantifying the (often small) proportion of total costs attributable to drugs expenditure, pharmaceutical companies seek to remind payers that it might be inappropriate to focus attention on cutting drugs expenditure. A disease management approach that considers total costs and benefits can be used to highlight the benefits of interventions (e.g. drug treatments) that impact on high cost elements of care, by, for example, reducing hospitalisation rates.

The advent of primary care trusts, which hold budgets to pay for the healthcare of their local communities in the UK, has created healthcare organisations that in many ways mimic HMOs. However, important differences remain (Koperski 2000). For instance, although managed care organisations in the US encourage primary care gatekeeping by family doctors, between one-third and one-half of patients still refer themselves directly to specialists (Forrest & Reid 1997).

Some disease management schemes have encompassed an element of risk sharing with healthcare payers or providers (an example is given in Box 5.1). A further example in the UK is the agreement reached with manufacturers of beta interferon in relation to health outcomes for patients with multiple

---

Box 5.1   The UK Outcomes Guarantee project

The UK now has a series of national guidelines and benchmarks of best practice known as National Service Frameworks. One of these is for coronary heart disease and has targets for the use of statins to lower cholesterol in patients with existing circulatory disease. The concern for the GPs and health service managers in the state-funded NHS is that there is currently insufficient infrastructure to implement and monitor these recommendations. The tendency could be to overprescribe, which would lead to enormous cost pressures – statins currently account for approximately 7% of the drugs budget.

One way of controlling the diffusion of new drugs is to set up an 'outcome guarantee' (Chapman et al 2003). This involves a pharmaceutical company and the key health service stakeholders (primary care and hospital trusts) agreeing on the outcomes they expect from a particular drug intervention. If the drug fails to fulfil expectations, the pharmaceutical company refunds the health service for the cost of the drug. This means that the company is encouraged to promote responsible prescribing to optimise their chance of success, and the health service ensures its resources are not wasted on ineffective treatments.

The pilot was run using lipid-lowering drugs for the following reasons:

- this is a high-priority treatment area
- there is a consensus on recommended practice and clear guidelines
- the treatment outcome is objective and measurable
- there is high local morbidity
- there was an interested pharmaceutical partner.

The outcome related to attaining an agreed target of less than 3 mmol/L for low-density lipids, and related to a total population – not individual patients. The steering group made an adjustment for patient non-compliance, which was based on the original clinical trials. Once the project had been approved by the local ethics committee it was readily accepted by GPs and taken up by all but one practice in the primary care trust.

---

sclerosis being treated with the drug. This is different to the US model, as all the manufacturers are involved and it is non-competitive. Payments to the companies manufacturing the drugs will be linked to outcomes. After a period of assessment, if the drug has cost-effective outcomes, payments will continue but if not, payments to the manufacturers will be reduced on a sliding scale (Liddell 2002, Mayor 2001).

In the US, many companies have entered into agreements to cover the cost of care for patients suffering from a given condition (so-called 'capitation' schemes). These arrangements mean that the companies concerned are effectively acting as insurers. The challenge for these companies is to be able to assess the financial consequences of different levels of risk. This has resulted in different models as companies respond to pressure to reduce prices to capitated populations (see Box 5.2).

Outside the US – in Western Europe, Canada and Australia, for example – disease management approaches tend to be much less driven by pharmaceutical company influences. In Western Europe the notion of 'shared care' can be seen as a precursor to formal disease management approaches. Whereas individual disease management schemes differ according to the disease and local context, in general, shared care can be understood in terms of the first steps in a move towards more integrated approaches to care. Shared care involves bringing together providers to create shared understanding of

---

Box 5.2   The Florida 'Healthy State' initiative

An innovative model has been piloted in Florida. Rather than offering rebates in exchange for placing drugs on the state's Medicaid formulary, Pfizer offered funding for 10 hospital systems to hire 55 'care managers' to work with Medicaid patients and recommend changes to their lifestyle and disease management. These included:

- diet, exercise, appropriate dosage of medication and smoking cessation
- giving patients the tools and education to monitor their health at home, e.g. weight scales, glucometers, peak flow meters and blood-pressure cuffs
- access to a 24-h, 7-day-a-week triage telephone line run by state-registered nurses.

The objective of the programme is to reduce hospital and doctor visits, and hence reduce costs by concentrating on helping patients manage costly diseases better (the initial focus was on asthma, diabetes and high blood pressure). Early successes have been:

- a reduction in the number of patients who did not monitor their blood sugar – from 21% to 5%
- increasing the use of peak flow meters from 12% to 50% of asthmatics.

The state anticipates that if the programme is fully successful it could save $33 million in one year.

---

linkages in care processes. In addition, the aim is to improve the quality of care by developing an understanding of the **perspectives** of patients and other caregivers in the system.

Generally, disease management approaches have gone beyond this to include the incorporation of formal guidelines for care and an increased emphasis on scrutinising the roles of those providing care. This shift can be conceived in terms of a move away from rules about the right and wrong ways of doing things and a redefinition of care in terms of 'doing the right things' (Vrijhoef et al 2001). Importantly, this has involved the questioning of traditional hierarchies and professional boundaries and the redefinition, in some cases of roles and responsibilities in an attempt to 'do the right things'.

In the UK, the extension of prescribing rights to nurses and pharmacists will open further opportunities; these 'supplementary prescribers' have to prescribe to agreed protocols. Thus, for the first time, primary care trusts have the opportunity to direct prescribing, which in turn raises the possibility of some form of capitation arrangement with pharmaceutical companies.

In summary, the rationale for disease management can be seen in terms of a number of factors. These include a desire to:

- contain costs
- improve health outcomes
- reduce variations in care
- improve the quality of care provided
- maintain or increase drug sales.

Cost containment is not necessarily the same thing as a cost-effective use of resources. Improvements in the quality of care might require additional resources. Third-party payers attempting to contain costs within annual budgets might be forced to choose between cost effectiveness and cost containment.

Pharmacoeconomics and disease management

Traditionally, pharmacoeconomic evaluation has been concerned with the costs and benefits of a drug treatment versus some relevant comparator. In the real world, where decision makers have to deal with health systems in the wider context, such an approach might be too narrow to be useful. In particular, an evaluation that suggests that drug A, although more expensive than drug B, is more cost effective, does not help decision makers who have to grapple with issues of **affordability** as well as value for money. One of the advantages of a disease management approach (in theory at least) is that by taking into account the coordination of resources across the healthcare system it is possible to consider any savings in one part of the system arising from increased expenditure elsewhere. For example, by spending more on improved management (drugs, monitoring, ambulatory care, etc.) in a non-hospital setting, it might be possible to reduce costs (fewer emergency admissions for patients with chronic disease) in another part of the system. By going beyond a narrow head-to-head comparison of two drugs, the application of **pharmacoeconomics** in a disease management context provides decision makers with a much richer picture from which to make choices. This approach also enables decision makers to identify savings that can be used to fund developments where it is cost effective to do so.

As our example from the US illustrates (see Box 5.2), one of the attractions of the disease management approach has been its ability to identify ways of redesigning care to improve quality within affordable limits. This has often been achieved by spending more in one sector and saving money elsewhere as a consequence. One of the advantages of pharmacoeconomics in the context of disease management is its ability to suggest a redeployment of existing resources to produce an affordable and more cost-effective form of service provision. However, in many instances affordability will still present a barrier to the adoption of disease management approaches. The example in Box 5.3 illustrates why this might be the case.

IMPLEMENTING DISEASE MANAGEMENT

Theory and practice

Disease management approaches are characterised by the existence of formal guidelines. The assumption behind the guidelines movement is that valid and reliable knowledge is to be obtained mainly from the accumulation of research conducted by experts according to strict criteria. Ideally, guidelines draw on data from randomised controlled trials (RCTs), which reflect probabilistic outcomes for 'average' or 'typical' – as opposed to individual – patients.

One issue with RCTs is the 'representativeness' of the patients recruited into the study. This is because the study objective is to evaluate the **efficacy**

Box 5.3 Adopting a disease management approach in the real world

Redesign and coordinate care
Let us suppose that we embark on a disease management exercise and examine the costs and benefits of alternative ways of coordinating what was previously a fragmented service. We identify changes that would result in a more cost-effective form of service provision by, for example, spending more on new drugs and better ambulatory care and less on inpatient care.

Quantify costs and benefits of changes
We spend £500 per patient but prevent one admission for every three patients treated under the new way of working. Each admission costs £3500, which means that we are saving £2000 for every three patients we manage in this way. In addition, there will probably be improved health outcomes – in terms of quality of life, for example.

Counting the costs of disease management in the real world
In practice, in a state-funded system like the UK NHS, if hospital admissions are reduced then having empty beds on wards will not release £3500 per admission prevented because much of this cost will be fixed and will only reduce with large reductions in volumes of activity (e.g. closing an entire ward, not just having one empty bed). Much of this saving will be notional in the sense that it will not be available to fund the improved services in a non-hospital setting.

Another problem in practice is that disease management might require investment now to produce savings in the future. Where decision makers are faced with annual budgets and short-term planning, it might not be possible in affordability terms to adopt a disease management approach, however desirable that might be.

and safety of a healthcare intervention. Clinical trial subjects therefore tend not to be typical of patients managed routinely in clinical practice. Evidence describing the resources and outcomes of typical patients managed (e.g. in the NHS) enables us to benchmark a specific condition in relation to other common conditions that invariably compete for our attention and resources.

The act of issuing clinical guidelines does not automatically result in their implementation. Guidelines might be resisted on the grounds that they reduce flexibility and limit clinical freedom. In addition, the lack of evidence on the **effectiveness** of healthcare interventions, particularly non-pharmaceutical interventions, has hampered the development of guidelines in many disease areas. In recognition of the problems of implementing guidelines, the UK National Service Frameworks (NSF) have been produced for major areas and disease groups to bring together the best evidence of clinical and cost effectiveness, with the views of service users, to determine the best ways of providing particular services. The implementation of NSF guidelines will be audited and clinicians who fail to implement them will be held to account.

For health economists, guidelines should incorporate not only evidence about what works but also available data on the cost effectiveness of treatment alternatives. For this reason, the economic evaluation of healthcare technologies has a potentially large contribution to make to disease management programmes within healthcare systems. Indeed, disease management programmes in the US are often sold to purchasers on the basis that costs will reduce or benefits increase or both.

The NSF approach to managing disease is less about cost containment – indeed, these standards are currently the major drivers of the increases in medicines expenditure in the UK at present – than improving quality, reducing inequalities and improving health outcomes. However, although the aims of the NSFs are laudable, in practice they could create problems for those involved in delivering care within limited resources. In addition, although outcome guarantee schemes of the kind described in Box 5.1 (p. 74) provide a practical means of ensuring that limited resources are used cost effectively, cost effectiveness does not address the issue of affordability.

Replacing fragmented and unsystematic care with better coordinated care might require additional resources, because a systematic approach might well identify more patients for treatment. Certainly, the evidence highlighting the extent of underprescribing for patients with coronary heart disease suggests that delivering optimal therapeutic regimens, as defined in the NSF, will increase expenditure. However, any savings in the longer term will not be immediately available to those charged with balancing annual budgets in the short term. In addition, although NSFs aim to bring together the best evidence on clinical and cost effectiveness, such evidence might be lacking, which means that expert opinion will be required as a substitute.

But who are the experts here? Policies such as the 'expert patient' programme in the UK aim to incorporate the experiences of chronically ill patients and to ensure that they become participants in the system and not just recipients of care. Even where evidence exists, incorporating different perspectives of various **stakeholders** represents a challenge to disease management approaches underpinned solely by RCT-driven protocols. What is important to patients might be less important to clinicians, and incorporating these conflicting values into clear clinical guidelines could be problematic. Programme budgeting and marginal analysis are economic tools intended to allow stakeholders to make resource allocation choices within the context of resource scarcity and multiple, and sometimes conflicting, perspectives. This is discussed in more detail below.

PROGRAMME BUDGETING AND MARGINAL ANALYSIS (PBMA)

Programme budgeting (PB) and marginal analysis (MA) are two different, but linked, activities.

PBMA combines these two elements and offers a framework that emphasises:

- use of local cost and activity data
- the availability of evidence on effectiveness
- an appreciation that many decisions are still based on value judgements but that the important thing is to be as open as possible about such judgements.

PBMA starts from the existing services and examines marginal changes in those services, rather than starting with a blank piece of paper and attempting to allocate resources in some hypothetical fashion.

Concept box 5.1 – Programmed budgeting (PB) and marginal analysis (MA)

The basic premise of PB is that it is important to understand how resources are currently spent before thinking about ways of changing this pattern of resource use.

The premise underlying MA is that to have more of some services it is necessary to have less of others or, if growth monies are available, that some projects will be funded whereas others will not. MA asks:

- If additional resources were allocated to this programme, how best could these be deployed to ensure the greatest possible increase in benefit?
- If resources for the programme are reduced, how best should these cuts be made to ensure the minimum loss of benefit from the programme?

The stages of PBMA

There are five stages in the PBMA framework:

1. Identification of a healthcare programme – usually based on a disease (e.g. cancers, coronary heart disease) or patient group (e.g. children, elderly).
2. Production of a statement of expenditure and activity by subprogrammes, i.e. the programme budget (e.g. by primary, secondary and tertiary healthcare).
3. Generation of a list of candidate services for expansion and reduction.
4. Measurement of the costs and benefits of proposed candidates for expansion and reduction, i.e. conduct marginal analysis.
5. Preparation of recommendations for purchasing.

The following summarises the advantages of the programme budgeting and marginal analysis approach to priority setting. PBMA:

- provides a systematic, analytical framework with which to approach healthcare priority setting.
- recognises that sacrifices are necessary to achieve desired expansion, i.e. if some services are to be expanded then others must be contracted in a budget-neutral setting.
- is a multidisciplinary approach to priority setting and can promote joint ownership of decisions.
- recognises the role of value judgements and subjectivity in healthcare provision and provides a means of making these explicit.
- fosters clear definition of healthcare services in the priority-setting process.
- fosters the setting of clear objectives for local healthcare services in the priority-setting process.

- uses locally relevant costs and (where possible) outcome information.
- breaks down the overall task of priority setting in the NHS into locally manageable tasks.

Problems and limitations of the PBMA approach

1. Local costs and activity. PBMA requires detailed information about local costs and activity levels because construction of programme budgets requires the organisation of costs and activity by sub-programme. This can be problematic because data might not be held at this level. For example, patients with heart disease who are seen in a general medical outpatient clinic might be recorded under 'general medicine' and not easily identifiable from aggregate data. Information in primary care might also be difficult to obtain, particularly where practices do not record all details of patient consultations. Financial information for inpatient care is likely to be based on hospital contracts, which might reflect historic service patterns rather than the true costs of current service provision.

2. Expenditure and activity. These do not always fall neatly into programme areas. Health treatments often spill over into a range of areas and services. Prescribing data is generally of good quality and available in detail but there might be problems in assigning drug expenditure to one programme. For example, diuretics prescribed to treat hypertension reduce the risk of stroke and coronary heart disease. Often the percentage split between programme areas will be an arbitrary decision.

3. Time constraints. PBMA takes time. The main constraints involve getting together a team that can meet regularly. Involving all stakeholders and sustaining interest for and commitment to the process can be a daunting task. PBMA is a multidisciplinary activity involving a range of players, including clinicians, finance, contracting and information staff. All of these have their own workload, which tends to be prioritised over the PBMA process. One or two motivated individuals must take responsibility for sustaining momentum or the process will flounder.

4. Extrapolating the costs. In practice, healthcare programmes come in 'lumps' and might not be neatly expandable or reducible. If we know the **marginal cost** of performing one more operation, we cannot assume that this can be used to calculate the additional cost of 10 or 100 more operations. Expanding an existing service might simply require additional investment at the margins, particularly if spare capacity exists. However, a small increase in activity could require a whole new theatre if there is no extra capacity in the current system.

5. Lack of evidence. The body of literature on the cost effectiveness of different healthcare interventions is growing. However, only a relatively small proportion of all services has been evaluated and the date, location, methodology and quality of economic evaluations vary. This means that any PBMA exercise will often be hampered during the marginal analysis stage through a lack of evidence of clinical effectiveness and cost effectiveness.

6. Marginal costs. Expanding a service at the margin might mean that we are now able to treat more patients. If these patients are at lower risk than the existing treatment group, the marginal benefits of treating healthier patients could be lower than for the initial treatment group.

7. The consequences of marginal changes. Although PBMA attempts to take account of the consequences of marginal changes in programme investments, it generally cannot look at all the 'ripple effects' of these changes. Some impact will be felt on other programme areas. For example, changes that keep people with heart disease alive for longer could increase the pool of people now at risk of stroke, which will influence the need for stroke services. Some impacts will be within the existing programme but will be difficult to anticipate or quantify. For example, a reduction in waiting times for an outpatient clinic might increase referrals from GPs, resulting in a longer waiting time overall and a drop in the threshold for referral, increasing the risk of inappropriate referrals.

In theory, then, PBMA represents a practical approach to allocating resources within disease areas to produce the maximum benefits. PBMA recognises that individuals and groups within the process will have different values and perspectives, but the aim is to bring people together to develop a shared understanding of the whole disease process and system of care underpinning it. The intention is that, by bringing people together, some sort of consensus can be achieved on the best way to allocate resources to achieve objectives.

Getting PBMA into practice

In practice, in addition to the technical problems of PBMA outlined above, other factors serve to limit its use. A further potential problem concerns the reconciliation of conflicting value judgements, or determining whose values are to count in the valuation process.

Part of the rationale for PBMA's 'expert group' phase is a recognition of the importance of obtaining consensus in relation to the value judgements, which inform the inputs to economic analysis. Such judgements include the:

- extent to which the selection of inputs is seen as valid
- areas seen as legitimate for scrutiny
- valuation of intangibles such as patient choice
- weighting of criteria for decision making.

However, although achieving consensus might allow economists to make progress when carrying out the analysis, it is important that those who are required to implement changes have some sense of ownership of the process.

In addition, in health systems that strongly discourage explicit **rationing** it might be difficult to disinvest from services. Clinicians might have more power in the decision process than those who commission care. Certainly, the public supports clinicians over bureaucrats in opinion polls and in this sense they can claim legitimacy for their actions, unlike health service managers, who have at best only weak legitimacy when it comes to disinvesting from existing services. Linked to this is the fact that those who commission care are often not in a position to issue commands to those who provide care. The move from hierarchical and top-down control to an emphasis on networks means that service changes must be negotiated. Even in top-down managed care environments in the US, attempts by HMOs to place maximum limits of length of stay have in many cases been thwarted by blocking legislation.

PBMA exercises have been conducted in England, Scotland, Wales, Australia, New Zealand, Ghana and, more recently, Canada. Despite its attractions, the evidence suggests that PBMA has not had a great impact on resource allocation decisions in health services globally. A recent international survey-based study by Mitton and Donaldson (2001) suggests that, overall across all countries, PBMA has had a 'positive impact' in 59% of 22 studies. Mitton and Donaldson note that because their survey respondents were the authors of PBMA papers, the results might present a more favourable view of PBMA than would have been obtained by surveying health services personnel. Additionally, 'positive impact' is defined in terms of setting priorities or shifting resources, and the former might refer to the statement of priorities in policy documents but with no resource shifts, the benefits obtained from these exercises are largely uncertain.

FUTURE DIRECTIONS AND CONCLUSIONS

A lot of hype surrounded the growth of disease management programmes involving pharmaceutical companies in the provision of healthcare in the US in the 1990s. However, it now seems clear that this sort of US-style approach involving provision of care is not being adopted on any widespread basis in other Western healthcare system at anything like the same pace. As one commentator has observed:

> The implementation of disease management in the USA looks increasingly like a particularly US solution to a US problem. (Pilnick et al 2001, p 762).

Disease management in the US tends to be associated with managed care. This involves cost containment and the promotion of effectiveness in a healthcare system characterised less by direct state provision or planning than via market mechanisms. Managed care in the US has largely not fulfilled its promise and may predict its demise. Although many European countries are not unsympathetic to market mechanisms, they do involve a much greater degree of state direction in the health sector. The expense of operating the sorts of detailed regulatory systems used in US disease management schemes is another factor that might discourage the adoption of such arrangements outside the US. Instead, existing providers and/or commissioners of care in many OECD countries (including Australia, the Netherlands, New Zealand and the UK) have developed disease management approaches more suited to their local context.

Having said all that, however, the question of whether such disease management approaches achieve their objectives remains largely unanswered. If disease management is to be adopted more widely, then more evidence needs to be made available in relation to actual, as opposed to potential, benefits. There is some limited evidence from the US that disease management reduces costs, but the evidence on effectiveness is mixed. There is a pressing need, therefore, for rigorous studies to evaluate disease management schemes. This represents a challenge that health economics, with its focus on the costs and benefits of care in the context of scarce resources, is well placed to take up. In addition, pharmacoeconomic analyses that assess the cost and benefits of new medicines are potentially useful inputs into the development of clinical guidelines that underpin the disease management approach. Because many existing guidelines focus on efficacy or effectiveness aimed at optimal care, with less emphasis on cost effectiveness, the challenge will be to develop disease management approaches that explicitly recognise the costs, as well as the benefits of redesigning health systems *ex ante* and then to evaluate these schemes following implementation to assess the extent to which potential costs and benefits occur in practice. The outcomes guarantee scheme described in this chapter recognises costs and benefits and offers an innovative means of ensuring that scarce resources are targeted at those who will benefit the most from them. Health economists will no doubt be watching its development with interest.

REFERENCES

Anderson G F 1997 In search of value: an international comparison of costs, access, and outcomes (OECD data). Health Affairs 16:163–171

Chapman S R, Reeve E, Rajaratnam G, Neary R 2003 Setting up an outcomes guarantee for pharmaceuticals: a novel approach to risk sharing in primary care. British Medical Journal 326:707–709

Fagan K 1998 Kaiser raising rates up to 11%. San Francisco Chronicle 31 March 1998:D1, D4

Forrest C B, Reid J R 1997 Passing the baton: HMOs' influence on referrals to speciality care. Health Affairs 16:157–162

Koperski M 2000 The state of primary care in the United States of America and lessons for primary care groups in the United Kingdom. British Journal of General Practice 50:319–322

Liddell R 2002 NHS to fund treatment for 10,000 patients with MS. British Medical Journal 324:316

Mayor S 2001 Health department fund interferon beta despite institute's ruling. British Medical Journal 323:1087

Mitton C, Donaldson C 2001 Twenty-five years of programme budgeting and marginal analysis in the health sector, 1974–1999. Journal of Health Service Research Policy 6(4):239–248

Pilnick A, Dingwall R, Starkey K 2001 Disease management: definitions, difficulties and future directions. Bulletin of the World Health Organization 79:755–763

Vrijhoef H J M, Spreeuwenberg C, Eijkelberg I M J G et al 2001 Adoption of disease management model for diabetes in the region of Maastricht. British Medical Journal 323:983–985

Cost of illness studies

6

INTRODUCTION

When we think about a patient's illness, we can define all kinds of 'costs', in the widest sense, that arise: the costs of treatment (medicines or hospitalisation), doctor's fees, and so on; these are all direct costs to the health service. There will be other direct costs to other budgets if the patient now claims sickness benefits and there might be further costs to society if the patient does not work and cannot easily be replaced, resulting in loss of productivity. Costs might also arise from a carer's time and loss of productivity, even if there is no actual payment for this, e.g. woman who doesn't work looking after her sick husband. Finally, there are **intangible costs** of suffering, loss of amenity, etc. Illness therefore places several burdens on individuals. But health policy makers have to assess the burden of an illness at a population level. The focus thus moves from an individual patient suffering from a particular disease to the burden which society suffers (in terms of disability, but also costs) from that disease.

A **'burden of illness'** (BoI; sometimes also called 'burden of disease') **study** aims to describe this. BoI studies are not economic evaluations – they do not measure the effect of an intervention – and nor do they examine marginal changes in the costs or outcomes of healthcare. They do not help decision makers use resources more efficiently, but rather describe the current levels of illness and the costs that arise from them, and the elements that make up this cost or burden. They are therefore closer to epidemiology than to true **health economics**.

Roles of a burden of illness study

Despite their flaws, BoI studies can be useful:

- They can describe the relative burden of different diseases and so be useful in helping to establish priorities for those health services in which it is possible that the burden could be alleviated, or where the burden is not adequately met.
- They can focus research on areas where healthcare expenditure is high or, for a pharmaceutical company, where the market is potentially large for a new product.

- They are also used by pharmaceutical companies who wish to emphasise the importance of a disease area in which they are going to launch a new product.
- They are valuable in establishing the baseline state (perhaps the 'do nothing' or standard care options) from which a proper health economic study can begin.
- They can clarify the real burden of some illnesses that do not feature strongly in traditional epidemiology in terms of their associated mortality or their demand on health service resources (e.g. migraine or chronic disabilities where a carer may lose time from work as well as the patient).

In making a case for a new product for the treatment of a particular disease, cost of illness studies are often embedded between the presentation of the epidemiological BoI and the presentation of health economic evaluations of the new product compared with existing methods of treatments for the disease. Such studies are often used to argue for more resources in a given area, and the implication that the current burden of a particular disease is large suggests this. However, a health economist would argue that BoI studies tell you almost nothing of value because they will not necessarily help you to use resources more efficiently.

COST OF ILLNESS

The term 'burden of illness' means different things to different people. Some public health studies describe – under the title BoI – the disease frequency in the population and the frequency and nature of complications, or symptom severity experienced by patients suffering from a disease in question. Other authors go beyond describing morbidity to also describing mortality from the disease. Still others describe all of these (mortality and morbidity), as well as resource use and costs associated with the disease. Sometimes the term 'burden of illness' is used synonymously with the term 'cost of illness' (CoI), although it is probably more helpful to think of the latter as a study focusing on the monetary burden, rather than the epidemiological burden, associated with a disease.

The differences between burden of illness studies and cost of illness studies lie in the measurements reported:

- a **burden of illness study** reports in terms of numbers of patients affected, bed days used or some other epidemiological end-point
- a **cost of illness study** usually translates all of the burden of resource use (measured as hospital days, physician visits, etc.) into monetary terms (by putting a unit cost to each element of the burden).

Of course, one cannot know the costs of an illness without knowing its burden first, so CoI follows on from BoI. How far one goes in measuring resource use will depend on the **perspective** adopted – health service, patient or societal – as it does in health economic studies (see Chapters 1 and 7).

Epidemiology

Many CoI studies involve large elements of epidemiology and the skills and tools of the epidemiologist. The key feature of epidemiology is the measurement of disease outcome in relation to a population at risk. It can be divided into two broad categories:

1. Descriptive epidemiology, in which the aim is to describe a disease or variable within a population or condition; it is this form that we are most concerned with in this chapter.
2. Analytic epidemiology, where the aim is to study the associations between diseases and other factors.

MEASURING BURDEN OF ILLNESS

Public health specialists have monitored the burden of some diseases for many decades, mostly in terms of mortality. The interest of such disease surveillance focused on the monitoring of any changes in the frequency, and the nature of the disease over time. Data on mortality or morbidity levels can also serve as outcome indicators at the population level, e.g. the UK National Service Frameworks outlined in Chapter 5 include such indicators based on mortality levels. More recently, projections of trends to predict future developments have become commonplace, thanks to available computing and statistical facilities and the relevant expertise. Problems of reporting mortality and morbidity data are illustrated in Box 6.1, p. 91.

Mortality

Mortality, i.e. the number of deaths, is one of the most basic types of epidemiological data used in BoI reports. This can be expressed as a crude death rate, the number of deaths in a given period (usually 1 year) per 1000 population at risk, or a specific mortality rate (i.e. the rate calculated within a specific population subgroup – often defined by age, sex and cause of death). For comparisons of mortality across different populations, standardisation (usually for age) can generate meaningful summary measures: the age-standardised rates, which adjust for the different age structures in comparison populations. Standardised life expectancy for different diseases, by age and gender, is often also available and valuable in conducting BoI studies.

Sources of mortality data

In many countries, mortality data are the best-quality 'health'-related data available. Notification is often required legally, and death is unlikely to be missed. However, in less developed countries even reliable death data are not universally available and one might have to accept a best-possible estimate. The measurement of mortality due to specific causes is potentially even more difficult as it depends on a reliable process of death certification, whereby the certifying doctor will have to report one or more causes of death.

Reliable death certification depends on reliable diagnoses, and these may be more or less subjective depending on the condition or syndrome in question. There are national trends in diagnosis – most patients who die in the UK with no clear other cause of death tend to be labelled as coronary heart disease.

Mortality alone is difficult to interpret in terms of disease burden, particularly that which is amenable to interventions. A useful indicator in that respect is the rate of 'potential years of life lost' (PYLLs). This indicator expresses premature mortality (in developed countries often reported as mortality before 70 or 75 years of age). PYLLs can be calculated for different causes of death; this allows us to identify diseases responsible for particularly large premature losses of life. For example, in the mid-1990s cancer was the main cause of premature mortality in women in many developed countries, whereas external causes (such as accidents or injuries) were responsible for a great proportion of premature mortality amongst men.

Mortality from different causes varies widely across the world. The World Health Organization (WHO) estimates that nearly one-fifth of global mortality is due to infectious and parasitic diseases (estimates for the year 2001). However, in WHO's African region (which excludes some North-African countries such as Egypt, Morocco, Sudan, Somalia, Tunisia), the estimate is 52%. In the same region, some 19% of all deaths in 1998 are estimated to have been due to HIV/Aids, compared with rates below 1% in high-income countries in Europe (0.3%) or the Americas (0.7%). This example is extreme but illustrates the point that mortality rates in one country or even one population within a country cannot automatically be assumed to apply to another.

Morbidity

Morbidity describes the occurrence of disease or disability in a population. Compared to mortality data, data on morbidity is comparatively limited in scope and quality. Morbidity is sometimes difficult to define, e.g. measurement scales might be needed and thresholds defined (and accurately applied!) for what constitutes clinical depression, hypertension or obesity for the purposes of clinical trials or for formal epidemiological studies. But these scales might not be used in clinical practice, where the diagnosis is often much looser.

Sources of morbidity data

The main sources of morbidity information include data on health service use for particular conditions (e.g. the numbers of hospital admissions or primary care consultations). However, health-service-use data can measure only that level of disease for which help is sought or treatments are available, and so might underrepresent the actual level of disease in the population because a large range of minor illnesses and chronic conditions associated with extensive distress and economic loss (e.g. upper respiratory tract infections, gastrointestinal problems, arthritic disorders, low back pain, some mental illness) do not present to the health service and so go unrecorded. This might be especially true for diseases for which no treatment is available, e.g. before the development of the triptans, the burden of migraine to the health service was very small compared to its societal burden because most patients did not bother to attend their doctor knowing there was often little that could be done to help them.

Population screening.   This provides another source of morbidity information for diseases for which comprehensive screening programmes exist. This systematic investigation of a whole population or a high-risk subpopulation to identify those who could benefit from treatment provides a basis on which to estimate the overall levels of the disease. For example, the UK operates national screening programmes for cervical and breast cancer. Again, not all women will take up those tests and many are not eligible because they do not fall within the target age groups.

Disease surveys.   Finally, specific epidemiological surveys might be available, and their data usable, for a CoI study of a particular disease. Morbidity surveys primarily measure the **prevalence** of a disease in a population. This is done by examining a sample of the population in detail; the methods of sample selection must ensure that the sample is representative of the population of interest. Cross-sectional surveys are limited to observations at one single point in time; they are thus descriptive, which is fine for establishing the prevalence of a disease. However, causal inferences are very hard to draw from them. This is somewhat easier in longitudinal surveys, which aim to make two or more comparable observations at different points in time.

 The UK conducts a 10-yearly national survey of morbidity determined in general practices and also regular health surveys of the general population.

Registry data.   For serious or chronic conditions (e.g. cancers, renal dialysis, cystic fibrosis, rheumatic conditions) registry systems exist that aim to record every occurrence of the disease and might also track the progress of each patient longitudinally. For instance, as part of quality assurance in UK general practice, it is a requirement that every practice sets up a disease register of conditions such as coronary heart disease. These can be collated to give good local epidemiological data and allow local planning of services. Some of these systems rely heavily on the cooperation of clinicians who diagnose and treat eligible patients, as well as on reliable and valid reporting mechanisms.

Computerised databases.   There are also ongoing systems for data collection from GP computer systems; these provide access to longitudinal anonymised patient records. However, there is often no validation of the diagnosis and

Concept box 6.2 – Prevalence

'Prevalence' describes the number of cases of a disease recorded in a population during a given period of time. The prevalence therefore describes the amount of a disease in a population and includes both new cases occurring during the study period and cases that occurred before this period but that have not yet recovered (it is often easy to think of the prevalence in terms of a pool of disease into which new cases fall). Prevalence is therefore always higher than the incidence unless the disease is very short. The term 'prevalence' is often used to designate a point prevalence, i.e. the rate of a disease in a population at a given time, e.g. prevalence of ischaemic heart disease in the British population is approximately 2%. This might also be known as point prevalence, i.e. the prevalence at a particular point in time rather than over a period.

only limited cross-checking of the completeness of the records. The best known and best validated of these in the UK is the General Practice Research Database (GPRD) from about 500 general practices: it is widely used, especially for drug safety studies. One of its great values is that it links the prescription of a drug to a particular diagnosis. Similar record-linkage databases exist in many US HMOs and elsewhere; they have a particular value in pharmacoeconomic studies because of the links between diagnosis, prescribing, resource utilisation and possible outcome.

Increasingly, such registries or clinical databases can be useful in pharmacoepidemiological and pharmacoeconomic research because – potentially – they provide a naturalistic picture of the course of the disease and treatment outcomes. However, to be able to determine the level of morbidity in the population, the registry or database has to cover all the population or at least a representative sample of it. It might indirectly permit estimates of morbidity levels of certain conditions, depending on the quality and completeness of the data and the representativeness of the sample (see Box 6.1).

Audit data. For cost of illness studies, particularly those that are intended to lead on to true economic evaluations of interventions, audit data, commonly collected in many health services, can be very useful. These describe typical pathways of patient care and outcomes and is extremely valuable where, for example, we might need to know how often a patient with condition X actually attends hospital, what investigations or monitoring are routinely done, and so on.

Aggregate measures of mortality and morbidity

To express the burden of disease in terms of premature mortality and disability, rather than mortality alone, various indicators have been compiled

Box 6.1   The problems of reporting morbidity and mortality

Figure 6.1 presents cancer incidence data, which shows much lower rates in Eastern European countries and countries of the former Soviet Union (the 'Newly Independent States') than in European Union countries. However, data on cancer mortality (Fig. 6.2) does not mirror this major difference seen in incidence (bearing in mind that deaths in some newly independent states are still underreported). The difference in incidence is almost certainly due to a large extent to the more detailed cancer registration procedures in Western countries.

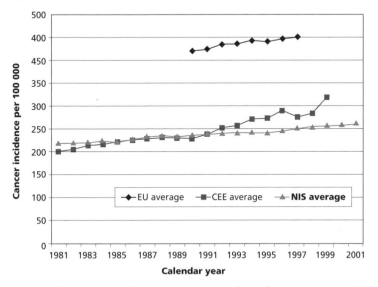

Fig 6.1   Trends in cancer incidence per 100 000 population for European Union (EU) countries, the newly independent states (NIS), and countries of Eastern Europe (CEE) 1981–2001 (from WHO 2003)

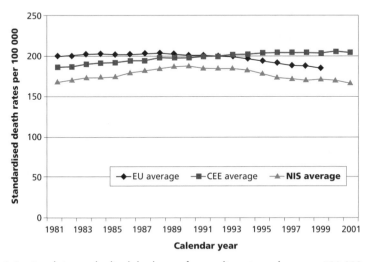

Fig 6.2   Trends in standardised death rates from malignant neoplasms per 100 000 population for European Union (EU) countries, the newly independent states (NIS) and countries of Eastern Europe (CEE) 1981–2001 (from WHO 2003)

**Box 6.2   Composite measures of morbidity and quality of life –
examples**

'In 1996, cardiovascular disease accounted for 22% of all disease burden in Australia.'
(Australian Bureau of Statistics 2002)

'... CVD [cardiovascular disease] is a major cause of DALYs lost in Established Market
Economies accounting for 19% of all DALYs lost. This is more than any cause apart from
neuro-psychiatric disorders. In Formerly Socialist Economies of Europe 23% of DALYs are
lost due to CVD – this is more than any other cause, including neuro-psychiatric disorders.'
(Murray & Lopez 1996)

'The *World Health Report 2002* estimates that 29% of all deaths in 2001 as well as 10%
of the total disease related burden, in terms of disability-adjusted life-year loss (DALY loss)
were attributable to CVD. This is, however much lower in WHO's African region (excludes
many Northern African countries), where it stands at 3%.' (WHO 2002)

from a combination of mortality and quality of life or morbidity data. After
all, policy makers will be looking for outcome measures of health gain, which
are comparable across different outcomes, and for indicators that clearly point
at areas of greatest possible health gain. However, such composite measures
are based on a range of assumptions about relative values of different states
of health or disability as well as – in the absence of relevant data – on
prevalence estimates of morbidity and quality of life themselves. They hide a
complexity of issues (for a description of the issues involved, see Murray et al
2000) but might be useful for regional or national comparisons (Box 6.2).

Examples of such composite indicators are healthy life expectancy (HALE),
disability-free life expectancy (DFLE), disability-adjusted life expectancy
(DALE) or years of healthy life (YHL). Similarly, disability-adjusted life-years
(DALY) have been developed to express premature mortality and disability
caused by a condition in a single measure. DALYs for a particular condition
take account of years of life lost and years lived with disability due to that
condition. This measure has been extensively used in recent WHO World
Health Reports because it is also a reflection of the economic burden of
disease, especially in developing countries.

RESOURCE USE

How does one translate simple descriptive epidemiological measures into a
measure of resource use? There might be summary data in some of the
databases examined already, for example, GPRD will track GP and hospital
visits and admissions, as well as drug use. One can then use the average cost
per GP visit or per outpatient visit or per admission. One could conduct a
more detailed examination of a representative sample of disease episodes to
explicitly record resource use in great detail, but this is very time consuming
and expensive. If the sample is representative of the population of interest,
results can be projected to that population and costs of the disease incurred

by the entire population presented. Some of the data required might be stored in administrative databases (e.g. number of hospital bed days for a particular procedure). Those who would undertake BoI studies must become expert at searching the medical literature, including the 'grey' sources (i.e. not peer reviewed, often not catalogued or easily found) where much of the data they need might well be found. This use of existing data is much less expensive than creating new data but where appropriate data do not exist, there is no option but to conduct an original study.

MEASURING COST OF ILLNESS

Assuming that we have good epidemiological data about the **incidence** and prevalence of a disease, and the resources used in the typical case of each episode of disease, there are then two broad options for how we measure the cost of an illness, based on either the prevalence or the incidence of a disease. Each has strengths and weaknesses:

- Prevalence-based costs estimate the direct and indirect economic burden to society incurred over a period of time (usually a year) as a result of the prevalence of the disease. This measures the costs over the defined period regardless of when the disease actually began. Most published CoI studies are of this type.
- Incidence-based costs usually measure the lifetime costs of a disease based on all cases with onset of disease within a given period. This is more demanding in terms of data but is also more useful because it provides a baseline against which new interventions can be judged. The incidence CoI study can therefore estimate the 'do nothing' or current care option in a health economic study. This is therefore probably the more useful of the two approaches because it can integrate with a planned programme of health economic evaluation whereas the prevalence study cannot be used in this way and largely stands alone.

Which is used depends on the aim of the study: if intended to be used for cost control or for bringing a disease to particular attention, then prevalence studies are more appropriate because this method identifies the major components of cost and can identify targets for possible economies. If,

---

Concept box 6.3 – Incidence

Incidence describes the number of new cases of a disease occurring in the population over a given period. An example would be the incidence of myocardial infarction which might be described for the general population or in a population with high cardiovascular risk. Chronic diseases also have an incidence, when the condition is first diagnosed.

however, the aim is to make decisions about which treatment to implement (i.e. to be part of an evaluation of alternative interventions), then the incidence approach is more appropriate because it will allow predictions about likely savings from programmes that might reduce incidence or improve outcomes. There is a trade-off, however, in that whereas the incidence study might be more useful, it will also be more expensive and time consuming to conduct.

COSTS

Costs as elsewhere in health economics can be:

- direct (directly for the illness, and often borne by a **third-party payer**)
- indirect (e.g. loss of earnings)
- intangible (e.g. pain, suffering).

CoI studies do not usually measure the intangible costs and can produce some bizarre results as a consequence. For instance, studies involving a heavy emphasis on **indirect costs** (e.g. loss of earnings) will not distinguish between a disease that causes death as opposed to disability preventing work; patients and their families put a greatly different value on each!

Measuring direct costs

Direct costs can seem relatively simple but there is sometimes a problem allocating the proportion of joint resources (e.g. in a hospital) that are allocated to a particular disease. This can result in double counting, with the result that the sum of direct costs for a range of illnesses can exceed the total expenditure on the health service. Sometimes, when a company or a clinician wishes to emphasise a point, this double counting of resource use is perhaps deliberate.

There is a range of possible sources for direct costs. One could either conduct a bottom-up costing exercise – minutely measuring resource utilisation in a small number of patients and putting a market price on each item – but this is very time consuming and expensive. Many studies use reference prices, and these are available for the UK NHS. It might be necessary to put together a number of different sources, for example, in the US one might take nursing home costs from the National Nursing Home Care Survey or physician charges from American Medical Association, each of which might have biases. Other studies use charges or prices rather than costs because these are easier to obtain and it might be argued reflect the market value of the care but, conversely, might also represent a large element of profit or reflect poor measurement. For instance, many hospitals in the UK NHS in the 1990s had widely different charges – even for simple operations – because they had never been costed properly. Many studies use a mixture of both reference and more specific measures of costs as appropriate.

It is worth remembering that because costs and patterns of care for common illnesses differ in different health systems, and over time even within the one health system, one must be very cautious in extrapolating a cost of illness study into any environment or time other than that in which it was originally measured.

Measuring indirect costs

As elsewhere in health economics, there is disagreement on how far one should go in considering indirect costs because there are both methodological and ethical problems. There have been two approaches to measurement of indirect costs, each with its own problems.

The human capital approach. When the person is regarded as producing a stream of output that can be valued at the person's earnings on the open market, then the 'value' of life is the discounted future earnings. Using this approach, the indirect morbidity costs are the mean daily earnings of the individual multiplied by the number of days lost from paid employment. Mortality costs are the product of the number of deaths from the disease and the expected value of the future lifetime earnings of the individual adjusted for life expectancy, gender, etc. and discounted appropriately.

This method has disadvantages:

- it leads to low values for those who are not economically active (e.g. the elderly and the very young)
- it ignores the psychosocial costs of illness – pain and suffering
- in any society with less than 100% employment, the loss of earnings to society when an individual dies or becomes disabled is temporary and partial because the lost worker is replaced within a short period by someone previously unemployed.

The classical **human capital approach** is now often considered inappropriate for these reasons and a refinement of it – the **friction approach** – which looks at actual lost productivity to society, is now thought better.

The friction approach. This acknowledges that if a worker is ill for anything other than the short term, another worker recruited from the pool of the unemployed will fill the post. Assuming that there is a pool of unemployed workers available then overall loss of production might therefore be no more than a few weeks. Society is indifferent to which worker gets wages and which gets social welfare support, although there is a substantial difference, of course, for each of the two workers involved. The true costs of the illness to society, therefore, are the transitional costs (sick pay for a period, costs of recruitment and training, and a transient loss of productivity). This approach leads to much lower indirect costs than the human capital approach, but seems more realistic.

The willingness to pay approach. Under this alternative, life is valued according to what individuals are willing to pay for a change that reduces the probability of death or illness (see Chapter 7). This approach is useful for indicating how individuals value life and health when deriving social preferences for public policy and in assessing the psychosocial or intangible burden of pain or suffering. However, it is influenced by ability to pay – high earners might be willing to pay more for their well-being than a low-paid workers simply because they have more disposable income.

There is an ethical issue here in that CoI studies with an emphasis on indirect costs might emphasise loss of earnings and focus on those of employable age or with high earning capacity, so undermining **equity** considerations (see Chapter 2).

Health service use of cost of illness studies

Health service purchasing organisations will be interested primarily in the demand on a variety of services caused by a particular disease in question. We have already pointed out that health service use is usually only a part of the actual level of disease in the population, because some patients might not have contact with services. Health service purchasers are most interested in the demand for their available resources (direct costs) and less in those faced by others (indirect costs). A CoI report therefore needs to make explicit whose costs it seeks to describe. Ideally, the perspective would be as wide as possible, not least because there might be knock-on effects impacting across organisational boundaries. For example, earlier discharges might use fewer hospital resources but cause an increase in demands for community services.

However, it is good practice to report direct and indirect costs as well as aggregated costs in CoI studies, just as it is in health economic studies. This allows the decision makers to judge for themselves the validity of the results and to decide what to consider.

In presenting health-service-use data, including the use of treatments, a local focus becomes very important. We need to know how a typical patient progresses through the different service areas, how long is spent in each and what variations this average picture might hide. Even if all hospitals in an area offer the same operation, there might be considerable variations in their accessibility and availability (e.g. waiting lists, variations in referrals from general practice), perhaps also in surgical technique and even outcomes. Some ability to localise a more general CoI study can therefore be very valuable.

Projections

As already mentioned, data on mortality, morbidity, treatment options and outcomes can lend themselves to being projected into the future. This is commonly done in incidence CoI studies. Such projections might be affected by a number of issues:

Demographic issues. Population ageing affects most countries – the number as well as the proportion of older people in the population is rising as life expectancy increases and birth rates fall. Therefore degenerative and chronic conditions will probably see a natural increase in prevalence (unless, of course, cures become available). However, older people are in general becoming healthier, with less morbidity at any given age.

Treatment methods. An increase in prevalence does not allow the automatic conclusion that resource use, complications, or even costs, will increase in proportion with prevalence, because treatment methods might change. Sometimes, for instance in health economic studies that focus on pharmaceuticals as alternatives to surgical treatments, a CoI study might fail to consider that the surgical treatment is not static but also progressing.

Risk-factor profile. Risk factors associated with a particular disease can change over time and, as the rate of exposure to a particular risk factor changes, so might the incidence and prevalence of the disease. For example, the prevalence of smoking has decreased in many Western populations and this has already impacted on rates of coronary heart disease.

Diagnostic categories. There are sometimes trends in the diagnosis of an illness arising from cultural trends or changes in definitions. For instance, the prevalence of hypertension is crucially dependent on the levels of blood pressure used to define this and can change as the recommendations from different expert bodies change. The rise in asthma over the past 10–15 years is in part the result of a greater readiness to make the diagnosis, as well as a probable change in the true prevalence. The increase in use of antidepressants has perhaps arisen not because more people are depressed but because the newer antidepressants were seen as a safe and effective treatment in milder cases.

KEY ISSUES IN CONDUCTING COST OF ILLNESS STUDIES

Some generic issues need to be considered when selecting and using data from other sources or studies for a CoI report; some have already been alluded to in the sections above, and we summarise them here:

Generalisability. The key question is: is the study whose data we want to use generalisable to the situation we are interested in? This question is much more difficult to answer for resource-use variables. Different health services treat patients with the same diagnosis in different ways, so CoI studies do not usually cross borders well.

It is important to pay careful attention to any inclusion or exclusion criteria used in such studies. The smaller the proportion of eligible patients who are included in the study and its analysis, the more concerned we have to be about the study's representativeness of its own parent population. However, this does not necessarily mean that the study findings should not be abstracted to a similarly restricted population.

A commonly occurring situation is that patients from one or several clinics or hospitals are included in a study; often these are more research-active centres, such as those affiliated with universities. But patients in such centres might be more severely ill than patients treated in smaller local centres because of selective referral of more severe cases.

Other variations are considered above including temporal or geographical variations in occurrence and progression of a disease, variations in risk and mediating factors, and variation in diagnosis or treatment.

Variables available. Studies using routine data are limited to what data are available. At times, variables in which we are interested might not be

Box 6.3   Example of a cost of illness study using only routine/secondary data (Stewart et al 2002)

From the abstract:
As hospital activity represents the major cost component of healthcare expenditure related to heart failure, this study evaluated the current cost of this syndrome to the National Health Service (NHS) in the UK. We applied contemporary estimates of healthcare activity associated with heart failure to the whole UK population on an age and sex-specific basis to calculate its cost to the NHS for the year 1995. Direct components of healthcare included in these estimates were hospital admissions associated with a principal diagnosis of heart failure, associated outpatient consultations, general practice consultations and prescribed drug therapy. We also calculated the cost of nursing home care following a primary heart failure admission and the cost of hospitalisations associated with a secondary diagnosis of heart failure. Adjusting for probable increases in hospital activity and the progressive ageing of the UK population, we have also projected the cost of heart failure to the NHS for the year 2000.

collected in the appropriate form. Similarly, factors of interest to us might not be available at all in the data source; or variables might be clearly defined but not meet our requirements. Inevitable omissions from a BoI or CoI study should be made clear to the reader.

Data quality.   Particularly if routine data or other secondary data are to be used as a basis for estimating costs of illness, the quality of that data needs to be known (Box 6.3). We have already seen that morbidity might be under-reported due to several factors. However, not just records, but also variables, might be incomplete in a data source. Thus, even if a representative sample is included in a study, but their treatments or deaths are insufficiently or incompletely reported, the validity of a study can be severely jeopardised.

One way of assessing the validity of measurements is to compare the data with that available in a different data source, which represents the '**gold standard**'. On large, professionally run data sources, such validations might already have been undertaken for different variables and many more checks of consistency, accuracy and completeness of data might be performed routinely.

KEY ISSUES IN REPORTING COST OF ILLNESS STUDIES

There is a major obligation on researchers to present the methods in considerable detail so that the reader can assess their accuracy and evaluate whether the results are relevant or not. Methods should describe:

- how morbidity and cost data were collected, including justifications of the appropriateness and quality of the data (especially if a secondary data source is used)
- the perspective – societal or health service?
- the discount rates used
- the reference years used and how recent the data are.

> **Box 6.4 Cost of illness studies – advantages and disadvantages**
>
> **Advantages**
> - Provide an indication of where healthcare efficiency might be improved by providing a league table of health problems according to their costs
> - Provide data to allow later economic evaluation
> - Raise consciousness of policy makers to particular diseases, making it more likely that resources will be deployed there in the future
> - Provide a single index of the burden of illness.
>
> **Disadvantages**
> - Assume 'value' of life is based on production or earnings – often no differentiation between death and chronic disability in this setting. Utility is ignored
> - Can distort priorities towards high earners and away from the more disadvantaged
> - Methodological problems about human capital approach
> - Can result in incorrect decisions because they look only at costs and not at costs and benefits
> - Risks of bias if methods or data poor or results not fully reported.

Results should:

- Report total and also disaggregated direct and indirect costs, to allow readers to make their own decisions on whether they should be aggregated. The costs often fall on separate budgets.
- Identify the different components of the direct costs so that the reader can identify where the burden falls, e.g. before 1990, the costs of schizophrenia often fell on institutionalisation. With a shift to new drugs and more active community care, this has changed. Similarly, costs of surgery fell on hospitalisation – new anaesthetic agents and streamlining of processes have allowed a growth in day-case surgery and now the anaesthetic agents consume a greater portion of the surgery budget.
- Include **sensitivity analysis**, especially where there are projections of future costs.

CONCLUSIONS

Despite their limitations, BoI and CoI studies are widely undertaken. There are many methodological pitfalls. The information they produce is limited and although they can be useful in drawing attention to an area, they do not define good use of resources. They must not be allowed to mislead decision makers into thinking that putting more money into a high-cost area is actually a good idea – a mistake that is sometimes made by politicians! Good studies can be valuable for decision makers if used properly – poor studies or poorly used studies can just cause problems. The advantages and disadvantages of cost of illness studies are summarised in Box 6.4.

REFERENCES

Australian Bureau of Statistics 2002 Australian Social Trends 2002: Health – mortality and morbidity. Cardiovascular disease: 20th century trends. Online. Available:

www.abs.gov.au/ausstats/abs@.nsf/94713ad445ff1425ca25682000192af2/4c9f3487e20b7 5caca256bcd008272f5!OpenDocument (accessed 2 December 2002)

Murray J L, Lopez A D 1996 In: Rayner M, Petersen S, eds. European cardiovascular disease statistics, 2000 edition. British Heart Foundation Health Promotion Research Group, Oxford. Online. Available: www.dphpc.ox.ac.uk/bhfhprg/stats/2000/europe/download/ europe.pdf (accessed 2 December 2002)

Murray C, Salomon J, Mathers C 2000 A critical examination of summary measures of population health. Bulletin of the World Health Organization 78(8):981–994

Stewart S, Jenkins A, Buchan S et al 2002 The current cost of heart failure to the National Health Service in the UK. European Journal of Heart Failure 4:361–371

World Health Organization (WHO) 2002 The World Health Report 2002: Reducing risks, promoting healthy life. WHO, Geneva. Online. Available: www.who.ch

World Health Organization (WHO) 2003 European 'Health for all' database. WHO Regional Office for Europe, Copenhagen

FURTHER READING

Coggon D, Rose G, Barker J 1997 Epidemiology for the uninitiated, 4th edn. BMJ Publishing, London

Drummond M 1992 Cost of illness studies: a major headache? Pharmacoeconomics 2:1–4

Rice D P 1994 Cost of illness studies – fact or fiction? Lancet 344:1519–1520

Approaches to pharmacoeconomic analysis

7

INTRODUCTION

This chapter explains the relation between **pharmacoeconomics**, economics and economic evaluation, exposing the economic concepts behind the different types of pharmacoeconomic evaluation used by analysts and illustrating their applicability to practical problems; in doing so, it covers the concepts that lay the foundations of economic analysis, in general, and pharmacoeconomic evaluation, in particular. The section entitled 'Costs in economic evaluation' (p. 103) presents the principles for the identification and valuation of costs in economic evaluation. The next section, 'Outcomes in pharmacoeconomics' (p. 107), highlights the distinctive elements of the different types of pharmacoeconomic evaluation. Next, the section 'Types of economic evaluation' (p. 108) explains in more detail each type of evaluation, noting their strengths and limitations. Key issues of methodological debate in pharmacoeconomics are the subject of the next two sections ('Dealing with time – discounting', p. 122 and 'Dealing with uncertainty – sensitivity analysis', p. 123), which discuss the valuation of costs and benefits that occur at different points in time and the available approaches to account for the effect of uncertainty on the results of pharmacoeconomic studies, respectively. The chapter ends with a summary of the material covered, a discussion of the situations where the different types of pharmacoeconomic studies are commonly used and the analytical complexities often faced. It is expected that, by the end of the chapter, the reader will be able to:

- discriminate between the types of pharmacoeconomic evaluation available
- discern the most appropriate study type to use in a given situation
- interpret the results arising from those studies.

As outlined in Chapter 1, economics is concerned with the allocation of resources in a world where resources are finite and wants are infinite. It is based on the premise of scarcity of resources (both financial and physical), implying that not everything that is desired can be acquired and that a choice must be made between competing uses of those limited resources. Thus, for example, when we are choosing a car, our desire for luxury and speed is restricted by our income. The decision of whether to buy an expensive car might be seen as a simple question of how much we want this car relative to the range of other potential uses for our money. If we end up buying a car, it is argued, we imply that the benefits of having a car are greater than the benefits provided by the goods that had to be sacrificed to pay for it. According to economic theory, provided that markets operate competitively, the price paid for the service or good in question is approximately equal to its value to purchasers and sellers.

Because perfect competition is unlikely to describe the situation of most markets for healthcare services, including that of pharmaceuticals, the prices paid by purchasers (e.g. the NHS in the UK or a **health maintenance organisation** [HMO] in the US) might not be an adequate benchmark for determining the benefits gained or forgone by individuals in society on whose behalf purchases are made, from the availability of a new technology or drug. This and other issues are addressed through the use of economic evaluation methods, in general, and pharmacoeconomics, in particular.

Economic evaluation is concerned with identifying, measuring and valuing inputs (i.e. estimating costs) and outputs (benefits) of programmes with the aim of determining whether these lead to a collective improvement in the welfare of individuals relative to the status quo (i.e. current normal practice). Thus, any economic evaluation compares a drug therapy with an alternative course of action or, if it is realistic, against 'doing nothing'. A collective improvement in welfare is characterised, in economic evaluation, as situations where the aggregate costs of a programme are less than the aggregate benefits it produces.

Because pharmacoeconomics is concerned with identifying healthcare therapies that represent an efficient use of scarce resources, a crucial question is, 'What is 'efficiency'?' Economists often distinguish between three types of efficiency, and the definition chosen will partly determine the pharmacoeconomic study type to use in a particular situation:

1. technical efficiency
2. production efficiency
3. allocative efficiency.

Technical efficiency. This describes a situation where no resources are wasted, for example, a patient taking a prescribed drug dosage achieves the highest therapeutic benefit possible for the given amount of drug provided.

Production efficiency. This extends the previous idea to the analysis of more than one input for treatment (e.g. amount of drug and nurse time required in prepare and administer a medication), so that a common unit to express resource utilisation is needed: it requires that the optimal therapeutic effect is achieved at the lowest cost.

Allocative efficiency. This is achieved when the choice of therapies is consistent with the objective of maximising the difference between benefits and costs (i.e. 'net benefits') across all areas of the purchaser's expenditure (e.g. public provision of services by the UK government) under existing resource constraints. We will see how the study types relate to these definitions later in the chapter.

Any pharmacoeconomic study should reflect the costs and benefits as perceived by a particular entity and any valid efficiency claims resulting refer to that viewpoint (i.e. the **perspective** of analysis). The analysis of efficiency can be as narrow as that relevant to a particular provider, like an HMO, or be broad enough to capture outcomes of importance to society at large. Often, the perspective adopted is that of the health system, with the aim to improve the allocation of healthcare resources within the healthcare sector. Such a perspective is acceptable if the impact of the changes in costs and benefits is largely contained within the healthcare sector. In certain circumstances, however, the impact of some healthcare initiatives are likely to range far outside the narrow confines of the health service and, in such circumstances, it is crucial that the economic analysis is equally broad (Box 7.1). In cases where healthcare initiatives place a significant resource burden on other public or private bodies, such burdens should be incorporated into the economic analysis.

The perspective taken by the pharmacoeconomic study determines the range of costs and benefits to be included. If decision makers in a health service are concerned only with the impact of an intervention on that health service then the analysis should still, where appropriate, identify and document major resource burdens that fall outside this narrow focus. By separately reporting results for the broad and narrow perspectives, decision makers are made aware of the implications of the therapy in question to their own purse, and at the same time are informed of the potential wider implications of their decisions.

COSTS IN ECONOMIC EVALUATION

The hallmark of economic evaluation is the inherent symmetry of its approach; it always considers both costs and health benefits. Irrespective of the type of economic evaluation used, costs are always measured in the same way. Costs could be defined as the value of the inputs of therapy, that is, the resources used to produce, distribute and consume, say, a new antiretroviral drug for Aids or a new pneumococcal vaccine.

A key concept in economic evaluation is **opportunity cost** – the value of the best alternative use of resources used in a healthcare intervention. For example, if your GP referred you to hospital for a scan, the time allocated to your care by a professional in the radiology department cannot be used for another person's scan and hence has a cost. If your appointment had not been made, and the radiologist did not have an alternative patient, then the cost of that radiologist's time is zero. In economics, the value of a resource or service is equal to the benefits derived by the consumer (the patient in the present

---

Box 7.1 Case example – migraine

The treatment of migraine may bring about important changes in resource use for the NHS as well as having an impact on the welfare of society through days of work lost to the disease by the working population. Any evaluation that only assessed changes in healthcare resource use may provide inappropriate policy guidance from a societal perspective given the limited nature of its focus.

context). For example, whereas the acquisition price of the drug is a questionable approximation to its alternative benefit lost from a societal perspective, it is certainly appropriate when considering the narrower perspective of, for example, a public health system.

Cost measurement in health economic evaluations follows three stages:

1. *Resource identification*: at this stage all the different resources consumed during the process of healthcare provision (GP visits, injections, drugs, diagnostic tests, etc.) have to be identified. Moreover, those resources whose utilisation is likely to change as a result of the clinical effects of the therapy are noted.
2. *Resource measurement*: in this stage, all resources have to be recorded in terms of quantities used (number of pills, number of staff hours required to provide treatment, etc.). The importance of resource measurement is that it shows you the true impact on the healthcare provision arising from the new service being evaluated. How many inpatient days are saved as a consequence of the onset of day surgery? How many more hours of operating theatre time are required? How many more doctors and nurses are required?
3. *Resource valuation*: this stage consists of applying unit costs to each element of resource consumption. In valuing resource utilisation, it is important to distinguish between costs that are variable, and thus likely to change as a result of the new therapy, and those that are fixed during the period of analysis. An example is the evaluation of a new, hypothetical, more effective chemotherapy for uncomplicated malaria treatment – call it drug X – that is being evaluated against sulfadoxine–pyrimethamine, the standard treatment in a given East African country. One of the expected consequences of the new therapy is a reduction in the need of patients for repeat visits to the health clinic because of treatment failure. To determine the cost implications of the new drug for the public health system, it is important to compare the additional cost of the drug versus the savings generated from the reduction in repeat visits, relative to standard therapy. A crucial question is then how to value such reduction. In other words, of all resource inputs needed to provide outpatient care (i.e. health professional's time, ancillary drugs, room space use, medical and diagnostic equipment, **overheads**, materials and supplies), which items would be saved as a result of the change in drug regimen? Unless the public health impact of the new drug is dramatic, the use of a more effective antimalarial drug is unlikely to cause a reduction in outpatient services in a magnitude that merits the closure of buildings, or a reduction in overheads (e.g. administrative staff time) and laboratory equipment.

Costs normally fall into one of three main categories:

- *Direct costs*: consumed as a result of the process of providing and seeking healthcare and treatment (e.g. medical and nursing time, drugs, inpatient days, outpatient visits). These costs most commonly refer only to those incurred by the formal healthcare sector, but occasionally also include costs to the community, social services, the household (e.g. out-of-pocket payments for travelling to the health centre) and informal care (e.g. unpaid care provided by relatives or friends).

- *Indirect costs*: generated in sectors other than healthcare. These include the costs to the rest of the economy (e.g. productivity gains and losses as a result of the process and outcomes of healthcare).
- *Intangible costs*: capture the social and psychic costs associated with treatment (e.g. anxiety, fear and discomfort associated with treatment provision). Because there is no obvious price or unit cost with which to value changes in these costs, pharmacoeconomic studies often do not include them in the cost estimation, but might report them alongside the cost results.

Resource identification

Part of the identification process consists of separating **capital costs** (items that are consumed over more than 1 year, such as vehicles, buildings, equipment) and recurrent costs (items that are consumed within 1 year, e.g. supplies, staff salaries and overheads – electricity, gas, water, food). This is important when, for example, the introduction of a new drug is associated with the adoption of new equipment needed to provide the treatment in emergency departments; in this case, the unit cost of the new therapy should include the cost of the drug plus a proportion of the replacement value (e.g. purchasing price) of the item.

Measuring resource utilisation

There are different ways of measuring resource utilisation, depending on whether it is possible to conduct a prospective evaluation of the therapy in question or whether only a retrospective assessment is feasible. Prospective cost measurement is normally constrained within the overall design of a wider study, as in economic assessments alongside randomised controlled trials (RCTs). Here, the analyst has to identify the events or outcomes that generate costs and, if possible, define the unit of measurement of such events. To illustrate, consider the case of patients with acute myocardial infarction (AMI) who are given early thrombolysis with one of two drugs being studied; among the differences in clinical outcomes between these drugs in RCTs are the **incidences** of cerebral haemorrhage, stroke and reinfarction. Often, the choice of units to measure events associated with resource utilisation is determined with safety and **efficacy** concerns in mind, and these decisions determine the level of detail of the cost study. The job of the analyst would then be to estimate the typical costs of each of those events. In any case, an ever-increasing number of economic evaluations use data from different sources (individual studies, literature reviews and opinion) combined in a model and available evidence on clinical end-points often requires assumptions on their likely resource implications.

Resource valuation

The final stage of a cost analysis involves valuing quantities of resources used as a result of a therapeutic intervention in monetary terms and aggregating across cost elements. Here, the unit cost for each resource element is multiplied by the respective quantities (e.g. drug treatments are multiplied by their acquisition price, the number of outpatient visits is multiplied by the cost of the GPs' time per consultation, the dispensing fee per prescription is used to value the number of prescriptions, an adverse event multiplied by the typical cost of its treatment). Two important issues have to be addressed at this point:

- capital costs
- joint costs.

Capital costs. These need to be calculated separately because they are inputs consumed over a period longer than 1 year. The standard accounting practice is to adjust the purchasing price to reflect the gradual decrease over time in the value of the future flow of services derived from using the item in question. We therefore annualise capital costs by using a standard formula that divides the purchasing price or replacement value of new equipment by the sum of a series of declining annual discount factors corresponding to its expected productive life time and an annual discount rate, usually that used by the Treasury or government finance department (Box 7.2).

Box 7.2   Case example – paramedical provision of thrombolysis

Take the case of an ambulance service for the prehospital provision of thrombolysis to patients with AMI. Among the costs to the NHS of providing such service is that resulting from the ambulance itself. The cost per patient of using the ambulance would be derived by calculating the annual cost of using the ambulance and dividing it by the annual patient workload. Assuming that the life time of the vehicle is 3 years, the annual cost of the vehicle is:

$$\text{Annual cost} = \frac{P}{1 + \dfrac{1}{(1+r)} + \dfrac{1}{(1+r)^2}}$$

where P is the purchasing price of the vehicle and r is the opportunity cost of capital investment per year. The value of r also depends on the perspective adopted. For example, the UK government currently recommends using a 6% rate to discount publicly financed capital investment. This formula can be extended for capital items with longer life times, with each additional year of life being associated with an additional $1/(1 + r)$ term raised to the power of the year number minus one, in the denominator.

Joint costs. Space and staff are often shared by different activities and a new therapy is likely to be associated with an increased amount of joint costs. For example, the same laboratory might be used for screening donated blood and the routine testing for HIV, so costs would have to be allocated to these services according to their relative use of the facility. In practice, this is done by one, or a combination, of the:

- relative use of floor space (the percentage of annual costs imputed is equal to the proportion of laboratory space occupied by each)
- relative number of tests
- relative amount of total time that the space is occupied in 1 year.

Once the above issues have been addressed, the total aggregate costs are calculated for each therapy under comparison. Total costs will include the cost of the therapy itself plus any additional costs of healthcare service utilisation; out-of-pocket costs incurred by patients, their relatives or friends and indirect costs from productivity losses from work. Analysts normally present these overall costs of therapy in the form of **average costs**, that is, the mean total cost per patient treated with a given therapy. However, to address the pharmacoeconomic question posed, results need to be presented as the **incremental costs** of the new therapy relative to the standard, (compare this with **marginal costs**, which refer to the additional costs incurred by expanding an existing activity by one unit).

OUTCOMES IN PHARMACOECONOMICS

The term 'benefits' in economic evaluation, refers to the therapeutic objectives that gave rise to the intervention and the extent to which the objective is achieved by each of the available therapeutic strategies. As mentioned before, all types of pharmacoeconomic study value costs in the same terms – typically in monetary units (e.g. £s or $s). Depending on the way benefits are measured, four types of economic evaluation study are distinguished by analysts:

- **cost minimisation analysis** (CMA)
- **cost effectiveness analysis** (CEA)
- **cost utility analysis** (CUA)
- **cost benefit analysis** (CBA).

CMA compares therapies solely on the basis of their costs, implicitly assuming that the health benefits between them are the same; CEA goes a step further and bases the comparison on a combination of costs and health benefits measured in natural units; a further refinement is introduced in CUA, which weights the effect of morbidity by the values individuals attach to health outcomes relative to their own valuation of perfect health and combines these weights with the amount of time spent in each state in an index of 'quality life'. CBA values health benefits in terms of money according to the individuals' strength of preference, as expressed in the form of their **willingness to pay** for health benefits.

Although the choice of study type depends on the objective or study question, there are occasions in which the analyst does not know in advance the type of study to conduct (whether CMA, CEA, CUA or CBA), and where she has to wait until the results of the **effectiveness** study are known to decide in favour of one or more types. Few pharmacoeconomic evaluations are presented in the CBA framework; most researchers focus on questions appropriate to CMA, CEA and CUA. CMA will be suited to address questions of technical efficiency and production efficiency under equivalent health outcomes; CEA/CUA are intended to respond to those of production efficiency while CBA is intended to inform issues of allocative efficiency.

Table 7.1 outlines how different types of economic evaluation studies differ with regard to the benefit measure and the way the results are presented.

TYPES OF ECONOMIC EVALUATION

Cost minimisation analysis

Cost minimisation analysis (CMA) is based on the assumption that the outcomes of two or more healthcare technologies being compared are equivalent and, therefore, the basis of comparison becomes cost alone. The results of a CMA, being the simplest form of economic evaluation, require little more than common sense to interpret. If drug X costs more than drug Y, yet is clinically equivalent, then clearly drug Y should be chosen. Using this simple decision rule, the optimal choice of drug can be made. A classic example related to pharmaceuticals is the case where a generic drug is compared with a branded drug. Provided that both are therapeutically equivalent, then a CMA is appropriate and, more often than not, the generic drug will prove to be substantially cheaper. The assumption of equivalence is particularly attractive

Table 7.1 Different methods of economic evaluation

Method of economic evaluation	Measurement of outcome (health benefits)	Synthesis of costs and benefits
Cost minimisation analysis	Assumed to be equivalent and can take any form (e.g. number of cases detected, reductions in cholesterol levels, years of life saved)	Additional costs of therapy A relative to B
Cost effectiveness analysis	Health benefits across therapies are measured in similar natural units	Cost per life year gained, cost per life saved, cost per patient cured, etc.
Cost utility analysis	Health benefits across therapies are valued in similar units based on individual preferences	Cost per QALY gained, cost per HYE gained
Cost benefit analysis	Measured in similar or different units and are always valued in monetary units (e.g. amount willing to pay to prevent a death, amount willing to pay to reduce exposure to a hazard)	Net benefits = Benefits minus costs, benefit–cost ratio = benefits/costs

in the case of pharmaceutical industry evaluations of 'me-too' drugs that tend to be bought on the basis of price rather than therapeutic effectiveness.

In practice, however, very few competing healthcare technologies are evaluated in studies that are powered to test for equivalent health outcomes. Unless the clinical trial on which the economic evaluation is based is set out to test equivalence, the use of CMA will be misleading and a simultaneous assessment of costs and health outcomes should be undertaken. Disregarding a statistically non-significant, but clinically significant, difference in health outcomes from two therapies can lead to the wrong decision if the drug or therapy with the higher mean benefit happens to be the one with the higher cost. Epidemiologists often caution against this form of misinterpretation by stressing that:

No evidence of effect is *not* evidence of no effect.

In general, the best practice is to combine cost and health benefit estimates into a summary measure and to describe the uncertainty of the new estimate by presenting its range of most likely values (Box 7.3).

Box 7.3   Cost minimisation analysis – example

In a multicentre, pragmatic, randomised controlled trial, McPherson and colleagues (2001) compared cerivastatin, a third-generation statin, with branded pravastatin for the treatment of adults with primary hypercholesterolaemia, 5% of whom had a history of previous coronary artery disease that had failed to respond to a dietary intervention. Primary-care doctors involved in the study were told to prescribe doses and titration schedules according to their normal practice. The study randomised 417 patients to one of the two treatment options and followed them for 1 year, measuring for efficacy, safety and cost outcomes.

The study found that the incidence of adverse events was similar between both trial/treatment arms (cerivastatin 73.6% and branded pravastatin 74.9%), the majority of which were mild or moderate. The primary outcome was defined as the proportion of patients achieving a reduction of at least 20% in their baseline low-density lipoprotein cholesterol (LDL-C) level after 1 year; the intention-to-treat analysis showed that this was achieved in 74.2% of cerivastatin patients and 74% of pravastatin patients. Given the observed equivalence in treatment outcomes, the authors decided to perform a cost minimisation analysis; this adopted the perspective of the third-party payer – in this case the Canadian Provincial Ministries of Health (MoH). The direct costs included in the analysis were those relating to drug costs (for the medications studied and those indicated for the treatment of hyperlipidaemia or for adverse events related to the study medication), doctor fees, laboratory costs and hospital outpatient procedures up until 1 year after enrolment.

Cerivastatin was found to be associated with total (direct) costs per patient of Can$1224, whereas the commercial pravastatin had a corresponding figure of Can$1452 – sadly, the price year was not given. Cerivastatin was therefore found to be cost saving (a difference of 228, 95% CI: 191 to 264, calculated from data reported by authors). The authors note that when the cost of generic rather that branded pravastatin is used (the generic became available only after the study was completed) the cost difference was no longer significant. They concluded that 'In this clinical trial designed to simulate a typical community practice, cerivastatin was as effective as branded pravastatin … in patients with hypercholesterolemia, but at a significantly lower costs' and that this '… was a reflection of the lower drug acquisition costs of cerivastatin compared with branded pravastatin'.

Please note that the examples shown in Box 7.3 and Box 7.5 is for illustrative purposes only. Cerivastatin was withdrawn from the world market in 2001 due to deaths attributed to rhabdomyolysis that led to kidney failure.

The more additional dimensions of health outcome are considered important for evaluation, the less likely it is that there will be evidence of equivalence between two or more competing therapies. For example, important differences in terms of quality of life can result from using two thrombolytics with the same survival benefit after AMI: analgesics are likely to vary in terms of pain reduction and different tranquillisers impose different side-effects. Even when comparing a generic drug with the same chemical formulation in a branded drug (where bioequivalence can reasonably be assumed), patients might express a preference for the branded drug. Only where strong evidence exists that two therapies produce equivalent health outcomes across all relevant dimensions of health can CMA legitimately be employed.

Once CMA, with its analytical simplicity, is ruled out as a basis for informing decisions to provide a therapy, the more complicated methods and decision rules for cost effectiveness, cost utility and cost benefit analyses apply. For one thing, both costs and benefits have to be considered in the decision rule.

Cost effectiveness analysis

Cost effectiveness analysis (CEA) compares different options aimed at achieving a common therapeutic goal. The distinctive characteristic of this study is that health benefits are measured in natural or 'physical' units, like reinfections avoided, additional patients cured, saved lives or life years gained.

The appropriateness of CEA for addressing a specific question such as 'does drug A represent good value for money?' depends on the answers to the question: 'Is there a single dimension of health outcome in terms of which the relative benefits of competing drug therapies can be measured?' Provided an affirmative answer applies to this question, the adequacy of outcome measures used in clinical studies (e.g. RCTs) to measure effectiveness will determine whether there is need for further longer-term studies or models in order to address the study question.

Once the adequacy of CEA as the framework for analysis has been established and a proper outcome measure has been decided upon, the benefits are combined with the costs in a cost effectiveness ratio. CEA would estimate the incremental cost per unit of effectiveness gained for the new drug relative to the standard that would provide clinicians with guidance concerning how much it costs to achieve an additional case free of the condition. This estimate is called the incremental cost effectiveness ratio (ICER) and its simple formula is presented in Box 7.4.

Box 7.4   The incremental cost effectiveness ratio

$$\text{Incremental cost effectiveness} = \frac{(\text{cost of drug A} - \text{cost of drug B})}{(\text{benefits of drug A} - \text{benefits of drug B})}$$

$$= \frac{\text{difference in costs (A} - \text{B})}{\text{difference in benefits (A} - \text{B})}$$

Incremental cost effectiveness ratios reveal the cost per unit of benefit of switching from one treatment option to an alternative treatment option, i.e. the extra cost per unit of extra outcome obtained with the alternative (e.g. 'cost per infection avoided', 'cost per cure', 'cost per life saved' or 'cost per life years saved' at a given point in time). This differs from the average cost effectiveness ratios, which reflect cost per unit of benefit independently of other treatments. The use of average cost effectiveness ratios to decide between competing treatments can lead to misleading results as they fail to acknowledge their mutually exclusive character.

The logical step following calculation of ICERs is to ask whether the more expensive (and more effective) treatment is cost effective. In other words, is the ICER for the given treatment smaller than the maximum amount that one is prepared to pay per unit of health benefit? In determining this maximum or ceiling ICER value it is common to refer to the ICERs reported in the literature for widely adopted interventions in similar diseases. An example of how this is done in the context of cost-utility studies is presented in the next section (pp. 112–118).

Four possible qualitative results arise in a CEA:

1. If costs are lower and health benefits higher for one drug relative to another, the former is said to dominate and would be the preferred treatment (Fig. 7.1, quadrant II).
2. The opposite case applies, i.e. the new drug is more expensive and less effective, and thus is considered inferior and not recommended for introduction (Fig. 7.1 quadrant IV).
3. Where the new drug is both more effective and more expensive than the standard (Fig. 7.1, quadrant I); on the basis of ICERs a judgement must be about whether the additional benefits are worth the extra costs of the new drug and, therefore, whether it is 'cost effective'. A threshold ICER value might then be used to define cost effectiveness.
4. As 3, but with the roles of the new and the standard therapies reversed (Fig. 7.1, quadrant III); the question now is whether the extra benefits provided by the standard therapy justify the additional costs of retaining it as the preferred treatment when the option of a new, cheaper but less effective drug exists.

After identifying the most cost-effective treatment option, consideration must be given to the question of whether this preferred option is affordable. In fact, restrictions because of **affordability** can result in the best therapeutic option not being implemented; pharmacoeconomic studies normally address this issue at the moment of interpreting and discussing the findings.

It is common for researchers conducting RCTs comparing two competing (i.e. mutually exclusive) drugs for the same disease to ask what cost per unit of benefit does one drug achieve, relative to the comparator, in terms of the trial's primary outcome. This research-friendliness of CEA often comes at the cost of making compromises in terms of the validity of the effectiveness measure: because RCTs very often have follow-ups that fall short of the time period needed to capture clinically significant patient outcomes, CEAs tend to

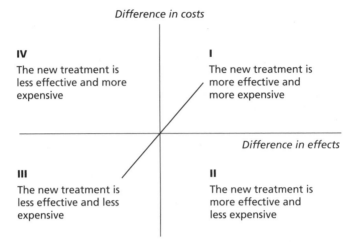

Fig 7.1 The four possible qualitative results in a cost effectiveness analysis

use surrogates or markers instead of proper effectiveness measures. An example is given in Box 7.5, in which the benefit of statins in secondary prevention of coronary heart disease (CHD) is approximated by the proportion of patients who achieved a recommended target low-density lipoprotein cholesterol (LDL-C) level at 1 year after the start of treatment; the basis for the choice of intermediate outcome measure was the accumulated evidence of a positive association between LDL-C levels and risk of CHD events and mortality.

Cost utility analysis (CUA)

It is worth noting that in addition to the clinical end-points normally used in drug trials, economic evaluations often incorporate a measure of quality of life. Such measures aim to assess the impact of the treatment on factors of greatest importance to the patient (e.g. pain, mobility and social performance). There are two different types of quality of life measures:

1. *Specific*: these instruments evaluate a series of health dimensions specific to a disease. For example, the Asthma TyPE questionnaire, assesses the effect of asthma on quality of life, the severity of common symptoms and distinguishes between extrinsic and intrinsic asthma.
2. *Generic*: these instruments can be used with any population. They generally cover quality-of-life questions and also questions on social, emotional and physical functioning, pain and self-care. Examples of generic measures include the Nottingham Health Profile, EQ-5D, SF36 and SF12.

Although in principle a CEA can be used to evaluate therapies designed to improve quality of life at a specific point in time (e.g. at 6 months after the

Box 7.5   Cost effectiveness analysis – example

MacLaine and Patel (2001) developed a decision-tree model (see Chapter 9 for a discussion of modelling techniques) to determine the cost effectiveness of the five statins licensed in the UK for lipid-lowering use, and to inform the choice of drug to be included in the formulary. The measure of effectiveness used was that of patients achieving an LDL-C level of 3 mmol/L at 12 months after the start of treatment, in accordance with the UK guidelines on primary and secondary prevention of coronary heart disease (CHD) and evidence on the relationship between cholesterol levels and the risk of CHD. A hypothetical cohort of patients with CHD managed in routine GP practices, and starting levels of LDL-C normally distributed around a mean of 4.37 mmol/L (0.71 SD), was considered for the analysis. The authors used estimates of efficacy in terms of mean percentage reduction in LDL-C from meta-analyses of RCT data. These estimates were converted into the corresponding proportion of patients achieving the target LDL-C level for each dose and drug in the basis of the distribution of initial levels. The model assumed 12-weekly monitoring visits at which the dose was increased if the target level was not achieved. Once achieved, the patient was assumed to remain on that dose and at the target level until the end of the year. The costs of GP visits and nurse consultations, drug acquisition, blood cholesterol tests and liver function tests were included in the analysis, which adopted the perspective of the NHS. Because the drugs were considered to be well tolerated and have similar adverse event profiles, the cost of such events was not included in the analysis. The authors reported the following results:

Statin	Treated patients achieving target LDL-C (%)	Mean annual cost/patient (£)	ICER £/patient achieving target
Atorvastatin	99.9	3721	383
Simvastatin	97.5	4086	431
Cerivastatin	67.1	3272	501
Fluvastatin	42.4	3382	820
Pravastatin	36.4	4296	1213

Source: taken from Table 3 in MacLaine and Patel (2001).

The table shows the competing statins ordered from the least effective (i.e. pravastatin) to the most effective (i.e. atorvastatin). First, note that the two drugs at the bottom, fluvastatin and pravastatin, can be ruled out as the drug of choice because they are more expensive and less effective than (i.e. they are dominated by) cerivastatin. Similarly, atorvastatin dominates simvastatin, and this leaves atorvastatin and cerivastatin for comparison; the ICER of the former relative to the latter can be shown to be £141 ([3721 – 3272]/[99.9 – 67.1]). This figure, and cerivastatin's ICER, suggest that atorvastatin dominates cerivastatin (by what is often referred to as *extended dominance*) because it is both more effective than cerivastatin and has a lower cost rate for the additional effectiveness achieved (£141 versus £501). This example describes a straightforward decision on the drug of choice on the basis of the study results; there are occasions in which the elimination process leaves two options, one of which is both more effective and has a *higher* cost rate for the additional effectiveness. This is when a decision on what drug to choose depends on the cost-effectiveness threshold.

start of therapy), more often the relevant question resides in the trade-off between quantity and quality of life, and in these circumstances CEA will not be a suitable framework. This leads us to the broader, more general framework of evaluation using cost utility analysis.

Cost utility analysis (CUA) combines the effects of an intervention in a more comprehensive way than cost effectiveness analysis because it measures both effects on morbidity (quality of life) and mortality (quantity of life) in a single preference-weighted index. The term 'utility' is derived from statements of preference by either patients or the general public in relation to possible health states. This type of study enables the comparison of different healthcare interventions, irrespective of the disease or condition. A range of methods has been developed to combine quality and quantity of life and to integrate these aspects of health across health states and individuals. The best known of these indices is the quality-adjusted life-year (QALY); in the QALY approach any health state of illness or disability is assigned a numerical score or 'utility' weight. QALYs are calculated by aggregating the number of days/years gained from a drug or healthcare intervention, weighted by a proportion that represents the relative value attached to the health state that the patient happened to fall into at the time. Results can be presented as cost per QALY gained or, strictly speaking, incremental cost per QALY gained (i.e., taking into account the costs and benefits of the competing intervention):

QALY = length of life × quality of life

The survival time in the QALY represents a 'hard' outcome measure in which patients can be dichotomised unambiguously between 'alive' and 'dead'. Although the extension of life can normally be considered a desirable outcome, survival of a patient who is bedridden and in constant pain provides very different levels of benefit per unit of time than survival of a patient who is pain free and experiences full mobility. A QALY calculation is presented in Box 7.6.

To obtain the quality of life weights or utility scores, health states have to be evaluated. Utility estimates can be obtained through direct measurement or by imputing them from the literature or expert opinion. The three methods of direct measurement that are most often used in economic evaluation are: **visual analogue scale** (VAS), **standard gamble** (SG) and **time trade-off** (TTO). These scales range from 0 representing death or the worst health state to 1 or 100 for full health or the best attainable health state.

Visual analogue scale. This technique requires individuals to state how they feel with respect to their health today using a 0 to 100 scale, for example using

---

Box 7.6   Calculating QALYs – a simple example

With treatment X
Estimated survival = 10 years
Estimated quality of life (relative to
  'perfect health') = 0.7
QALYs = (10 × 0.7) = 7.0

Without treatment X
Estimated survival = 5 years
Estimated quality of life (relative to
  'perfect health') = 0.5
QALYs = (5 × 0.5) = 2.5

QALY gain from treatment X = 7 - 2. 5 = 4.5 QALYs

If the cost of treatment X is £18 000, then the cost per QALY is £4000 per QALY (£18 000 divided between 4.5 additional QALYs).

a thermometer ranging from 0 (worst imaginable health state) to 100 (best imaginable health state).

Standard gamble. This technique involves assessing the level of risk that an individual is willing to incur for getting a better health state. For example a participant with osteoporosis might be asked to choose between:

- Strategy 1: without the drugs – to live for the next 20 years with mild pain followed by death
- Strategy 2: to receive a new drug for osteoporosis, if it had an associated risk of 95% of chance of recovery to full health for the next 20 years followed by death and a 5% risk of sudden death.

The score is obtained by varying the level of risk until the participant is indifferent to the two strategies; note that for both strategies the number of years is the same. In this example, the utility of living with mild pain until death is equal to 1 minus the risk of sudden death at the point of indifference.

Time trade-off. This technique involves asking respondents if they would be willing to trade-off time for an improved health state. For example, they are asked if they would be willing to take a drug if doing so made them completely healthy but shortened their life by 2 years. The numbers of years are then varied until the respondent is indifferent.

An alternative to QALYs are 'healthy years equivalents' (HYEs). This approach differs from that of QALYs in that HYEs measure all the different health states that an individual might experience as a result of a disease, rather than asking about a limited subset of health states. This aspect of the technique complicates its use enormously, adding extra burden to the respondent and the interviewer.

Another outcome measure that is often used to combine morbidity and mortality in a single index is the disability-adjusted life-year (DALY). Although this technique accounts for diminished quality of life from disability, its implicit valuation of morbidity is not based on individual preferences.

The difficulties of cost utility analysis arise, first, in conceptualising, measuring and obtaining comparative valuations of different levels of quality of life. Who should make such valuations and on what basis? For example, who has the 'right' to specify that 1 year spent in a wheelchair is 'worth' 9 months spent with full mobility? On what basis are such calculations made? A second problem with cost utility in general, and QALYs in particular, relates to the problem of aggregating estimates of QALYs across individuals: is a QALY gained worth the same regardless of the age, sex, education and sociodemographic characteristics of the beneficiary?

Similarly to CMA and CEA, CUA deals with mutually exclusive interventions. Given the way benefits are summarised (i.e. in 'natural' units –life years gained adjusted for the relative value to society or the patient of their associated quality of life) its decision rules are the same as those presented in Fig. 7.1 for CEA. In particular, how the results of a CUA or a CEA evaluation are interpreted might depend critically on the maximum cost rate at which it is deemed acceptable to derive benefits from more effective but more costly drug therapies. In other words, the choice of preferred drug will depend on the maximum amount that society or the decision maker is willing to pay for an additional unit of benefit.

An advantage of using CUA over the more restrictive CMA and CEA studies is that it permits comparisons to be made with other independent healthcare programmes or drugs, something which the first two types of study do not allow (Box 7.7). For example, questions such as 'Is simvastatin cost effective relative to pravastatin for the management of coronary heart disease?' or 'What is the most cost-effective treatment for migraine?' can benefit from using QALYs because a wider reference for establishing cost effectiveness standards (i.e. the maximum amount of money that a decision maker is willing to pay for an additional unit of benefit) can be used in the form of QALY league tables. This is precisely the topic of the next section.

Box 7.7 Cost utility analysis – example

In a study of docetaxel versus paclitaxel for the treatment of patients with recurrent anthracycline-resistant metastatic breast cancer, Hutton and colleagues (Hutton et al 1996, Brown et al 2001) developed a decision analysis model to represent the disease progression and expected costs of a cohort of patients. Although no standard second-line drug existed for patients with locally advanced or metastatic breast cancer, the authors noted that a third newly licensed option in the UK, vinorelbine, tended to be used on the basis of its lower acquisition cost (docetaxel, £1150, paclitaxel £1122, vinorelbine £441; figures in 1999 prices per 3-week course). The model covered costs incurred during the first 3 years from the start of salvage therapy and included, in addition to second-line drugs, the cost of a hospital day, GP consultations, specialist consultations, chemotherapy administration at an outpatient clinic, the cost of therapy in each health state (early progressive, late progressive, stable and terminal disease) and toxic effects (neutropenia, severe neurotoxicity and severe oedema).

A critical issue in advanced breast cancer is the effect that the disease has on the quality of life of patients. Given the lack of evidence on patient preferences for health states from the Phase III trials used to populate the model, utility values were derived from interviews with 30 oncology nurses from specialist cancer centres in the UK. The interviewees were questioned (using the standard gamble method) to provide rankings of health states on behalf of patients. The study results, for the base case where life expectancy differences in the model were used, showed that the total cost per patient for docetaxel was £1995 more than that of paclitaxel and £3594 higher than that of vinorelbine (figures at 1997–98 prices). The respective figures for the QALYs differences were 0.0862 and 0.2525. The incremental cost per QALY gained by docetaxel against paclitaxel was therefore £1995 and that for docetaxel versus vinorelbine was £14 055. On the basis of a cost per QALY value of between £20 000 and £30 000 presumably defining the threshold for cost effectiveness of the National Institute for Clinical Excellence, the authors concluded that '... docetaxel provided greater utility benefits than paclitaxel or vinorelbine at slightly higher additional costs. The results of our study support the use of docetaxel in the management of advanced breast cancer' (Brown et al 2001).

QALY league tables

When resources are scarce, priority setting is important to allocate the limited budgets to the most desirable healthcare programmes. In a QALY league table, different programmes are ranked accordingly to their cost per QALY ratio, and funds allocated progressively to programmes on an ascending order of the marginal cost per QALY rank until the available budget is exhausted. However, few countries have such league tables and, even when a serious attempt at using this approach in decision making was made, serious ethical issues limited its applicability, as the Oregon experiment shows (see 'Economic evaluation and decision making in practice', Chapter 3, p. 48).

To understand the informational value of league tables, a distinction must be made between programmes that are completely independent (e.g. the use of taxanes for breast cancer versus laser eye refractive surgery) and those that are mutually exclusive (e.g. simvastatin versus pravastatin for hypercholesterolaemia). Choice between independent programmes requires only the calculation of QALYs ratios, together with total allocated budget. Ratios are computed and ranked from lowest to highest. Those interventions associated with lower ratios should be prioritised over those with higher cost effectiveness (QALY) ratios, within the budgetary constraints. Consider the examples presented in Table 7.2. Ranking these independent interventions according to their cost utility ratios puts the combinational therapy (interferon alpha plus ribavirin) for chronic hepatitis C infection at the top of the list. According to the CUA, this is the most attractive intervention and should be given priority over the others. To decide which interventions to implement, however, the extent of resources available must be considered. Say the total budget available was £50000, then the most cost effective allocation of resources would be to implement the hepatitis C treatment until either all patients requiring treatment were given it, or until the £50000 is exhausted. If £100000 were available, all hepatitis C treatment should be implemented, then as much obesity treatment as the budget allows, and so on.

A league table must be:

- comprehensive: it should include confidence intervals, full details of intervention, target population
- consistent: costs should relate to the same year, studies should all be conducted in the country of interest
- credible: based on a high-quality evaluation
- updated regularly so that no new interventions or updated evidence is overlooked.

Table 7.2 Independent interventions ranked according to their cost utility ratios

Interventions	Costs (per patient)	Health effect (e.g. QALYs gained)	Cost utility ratio (per QALY gained)
Interferon alpha and ribavirin for chronic hepatitis C	£5930	13.78	£430
Orlistat™ for obesity	£734	0.016	£45 881
Riluzole™ for motor neuron syndrome	£5200	0.09	£58 000

Cost benefit analysis

In cost benefit analysis (CBA), benefits are valued in the same unit as costs, that is, in monetary units as opposed to natural units or QALYs. CBA has been used to evaluate therapies with outcomes that are difficult to measure with the conventional tool of CEA, for example, patient satisfaction with drug therapy. Although CBA is a theoretically and politically appealing tool, it also faces tremendous obstacles in implementation. As will be described shortly, conceptual difficulties in assigning monetary values to the process and outcomes of care can obscure the interpretation of the resulting values.

There are three different approaches for measuring benefits within CBA:

1. **human capital approach** (HCA)
2. **'revealed preference'** benefit measures
3. **'stated preference'** measures – contingent valuation and discrete choice modelling (sometimes referred to as conjoint analysis).

The major difference between these is that the last two reflect the preferences of individuals for health outcomes whereas the first approach is based on the market value of work contingent on such outcomes. These general approaches and their methods are described below.

Human capital approach (HCA)

This approach values the benefits of avoiding a premature death or disease by measuring the lost productivity from work as a result of such negative event. For a given individual whose life is spared, this technique imputes a benefit equal to the typical gross earnings accrued to people of the same age and sex over the years of life saved; in other words, the value of a saved life is equal to the earnings potential saved with it (see Chapter 6).

The role of HCA in pharmacoeconomics and outcomes research is now mostly limited to serve as a rough lower bound on the estimate of willingness to pay for therapies. Although it describes the costs to society of avoidable death or disabling disease, it fails to account for benefits other than those that are derived from the productive market activities lost to death or disabling disease.

Valuing health outcomes according to individual preferences is considered the theoretically sound approach for cost benefit analysis. There are, however, different methods to elicit these values, which are covered briefly in the following sections.

Revealed preference

This method infers the benefits of a transaction to an individual by observing the choices he or she makes in terms of risk and return when buying or selling goods or services in the market. A substantial amount of work on the value of a life has been conducted by analysing the occupational choices of individuals in relation to job characteristics such as pay and exposure to risks. This method uses regression analysis to control for differences in sociodemographic and geographical characteristics between individuals and to estimate the average rate at which individuals implicitly trade an increased risk of death while on the job for an additional salary. The difficulty in assessing the specific factors that influence people's choices and the practical inability to account for the value attached to the process of care itself are the most important disadvantages of this method, which is seldom used in pharmacoeconomics.

Stated preference – contingent valuation (CV)

This method constructs a hypothetical market for the healthcare intervention in question by asking a respondent to state the maximum amount of money he or she would be willing to pay for having the healthcare intervention, or the minimum amount acceptable in compensation for being denied access to it. CV allows patients, or carers on behalf of patients (and in some cases the general public), to indicate the intensity of their preference through their willingness to pay (WTP) to obtain the therapy (or, less commonly, their willingness to accept [WTA] compensation for not having it). The main weakness of CV is the difficulty in recreating a real-life situation so that respondents can prove their willingness to pay for a particular intervention. Another issue, rather methodological, relates to the negative implications that the link between WTP and ability to pay has for basic notions of **equity**. This criticism – namely that it is unethical to base decisions on people's expressed WTP because the preferences of poorer people will be attached a lower weight than those of rich people – are addressed by the technique so that 'wealth effects' are removed, at least to some extent.

Various survey designs are available for CV studies. One option is to use open-ended questions that explain the purpose of the survey question (i.e. obtain the value to an individual of a drug therapy for a specific disease). Respondents (in most cases the patient or a carer of young children or elderly patients) are then presented with a hypothetical scenario in which they have to pay for the treatment and, where a fixed fee is paid for treatment, might be given a reference value such as the amount of money currently paid per month for any prescription charges. The question is then phrased in the following terms:

> What is the highest amount you would be prepared to pay per year in the form of prescription charges for your current treatment? Answer: £ ...... per month

This type of survey question (and other standard questions on social class/socioeconomic status) is used in telephone or postal surveys or face-to-face interviews. Because high non-response rates can be a problem, aids are sometimes used whereby a respondent is presented with WTP values; the individual might be asked to choose from a range of values or simply to accept or reject any initial and subsequent auction-type bids, which are raised or lowered depending on the previous response, until the maximum WTP is reached.

Because the open-ended format is associated with problems of non-response and starting-point bias in bidding games, a popular option is the use of a binary 'yes/no' format where the respondent is presented with the same information as above but the question itself is phrased in terms such as:

> Would you continue your current treatment for, say, insomnia, if your payment for receiving treatment increased to £10 per month (tick one)?
> Answer: __ Yes __ No

A respondent who ticks 'no' is assumed to have a maximum WTP less than the bid, whereas one who replies 'yes' is assumed be the opposite case. By dividing the sample of respondents into subgroups according to the bid given, the relation between the price and the proportion of respondents likely to pay the price and use the treatment is obtained. This aggregate demand curve is used to derive the mean and median WTP in the sample, where the former is the area under the curve and the latter is the point at which 50% of patients responded 'yes' to the question. A common practice is to use regression analysis to adjust for differences in factors other than the price that affect a decision on whether to use or not to use the therapy.

The binary-choice format addresses the problem of starting-point bias in CV because it presents the patient with only one bid. In addition, it resembles a market environment in that it asks the individual to accept ('buy') or reject ('not buy') the drug, thus presenting the question in more familiar terms.

Stated preference – discrete choice modelling (SPDCM) (conjoint analysis)

Yet another technique for deriving WTP values using hypothetical questions asks patients or individuals whether they would use a new drug with certain characteristics – characteristics such as the cost, side-effects, effectiveness and frequency of the drug intake are variables believed to influence patient preferences for treatment. The same individual is asked a series of similar questions where the values of variables are changed and the resulting data for a sample of individuals are analysed using regression analysis for discrete data (e.g. logistic regression) to obtain mean WTP values for the sample. Very few examples of this technique, sometimes referred to as conjoint analysis, exist in pharamacoeconomics, although its use is likely to become more popular now that recent progress in computing capabilities has made the statistical methods easier to implement. A valuable advantage of this over the stated preference techniques previously discussed is that it can be extended to comparisons of more than two options. Thus, instead of presenting the individual with an all or nothing (yes/no) option, a range of options are presented, thus better resembling the market environment.

Having covered the different types methods in CBA it is now time to explain how the information obtained through them is used, in combination with the results from the respective costs analysis, to arrive at conclusions on the preferred therapy or programme.

Consider the improbable scenario of independent programmes – programmes that serve different purposes, for example, a new coronary care unit versus a new renal unit, and no fixed budget – where there is sufficient money to pay for all programmes! The net benefit rule states that if (and only if) the benefits of that programme exceed the costs, then the programme should be adopted. It naturally follows that if the costs were to exceed the benefits, then the programme should be rejected.

What if a choice has to be made between more than one mutually exclusive programme (see Box 7.8 for a published example), which serve the same purpose, and what if implementing one programme means the other cannot be implemented, or where the implementation of one affects the costs and benefits of the other (e.g. a range of competing Private Finance Initiative [PFI]-financed hospital contracts)? How can one decide between such programmes? Table 7.3 presents four mutually exclusive programmes. Columns 2 and 3 list the costs and benefits of each programme. For programmes A, C and D, it is clear that the benefits are greater than the costs. Column 4 confirms this because the net benefit (column 3 minus column 2) yields positive values greater than zero for these programmes. Note that programme B produces a net negative benefit and should not be adopted. The *net benefit rule* states that the programme with the greatest net benefit (A) should be chosen.

An alternative rule to the net benefit rule is the *benefit/cost ratio criterion*. Benefit/cost ratios are calculated by simply dividing the benefit (monetary units) by the costs associated with that programme – column 5 in Table 7.3. When considering a single programme, adoption must be logical if the ratio is greater than 1 (in this case A, C and D, as before). For mutually exclusive programmes, unless the projects are of the same scale and the relationship between benefits and cost is the same no matter what the scale of the projects are, this rule should not be used because it could result in different, erroneous results. The net benefit rule is the correct criterion in these circumstances. An example is given in Table 7.3 where the project where the most favourable benefit/cost ratio (C) is not the one that achieves the greatest net benefits (A is the optimal choice). To rank independent programmes, start from the highest benefit/cost ratio and work to the lowest: accept all with a ratio greater than 1.

Box 7.8   Example of cost benefit analysis

For diabetes mellitus, a new biosynthetic – Insulin Lispro – was compared with neutral insulin in terms of the willingness to pay (WTP) of participants in an Australian study (Davey et al 1998). According to commentators (Dunn & Plosker 2002), CEA or CUA is not suitable to analyse a new drug such as Insulin Lispro because utilities can be insensitive to clinical benefits such as increased patient convenience and reduced risk of nocturnal hypoglycaemia. A contingent valuation (CV) survey found that 76 patients (92%) preferred Insulin Lispro and that 7 patients (8%) preferred neutral insulin. In the analysis of WTP, the mean average incremental benefit per patient per month with Insulin Lispro was Aus$37.68 (95% CI, Aus$27.52–47.84). The annual cost of treating a patient with neutral insulin was Aus$197.88 and with Insulin Lispro Aus$268.20, resulting in an incremental cost per year of Aus$70.32. Cost and benefits were combined using a net benefit approach (incremental WTP benefits minus incremental costs). The net benefit of neutral insulin over Insulin Lispro was Aus$381.84 (unfortunately, the price year was not stated). This study showed that costs were exceeded by the benefits, supporting the case for the inclusion of Insulin Lispro in Australian formularies.

Table 7.3   Four mutually exclusive healthcare programmes – how to choose between them?

Programme	Costs	Benefits	Net benefit	Benefits/costs
A	100	200	100	2.0
B	90	60	–30	0.67
C	50	120	70	2.4
D	55	120	65	2.18

A third decision rule, called the *internal rate of return*, is often used to evaluate financial projects. This method consists of presenting results in terms of the discount rate (see the next section, 'Dealing with time – discounting') in which the costs and benefits of a drug therapy with long-term consequences (i.e. beyond 1 year after the beginning of therapy) are equal (see also the section 'Dealing with uncertainty – sensitivity analysis', p. 123). However, this criterion is of very limited applicability (given the short-time frame of analysis of many studies) and of little or no informational value in pharmacoeconomics.

Now consider a more realistic framework of a constrained budget. Decisions and decision rules under such circumstances are far more difficult. For single programmes, the fact that benefits exceed the costs is insufficient. Instead, a programme can only be accepted (based on the net benefit rule) if the net benefit exceeds that of the displaced programme. For ranking independent programmes or choosing between mutually exclusive programmes, neither the net benefit nor the benefit/cost criteria rules apply. Instead, solutions must be obtained by more complex means, such as by linear or dynamic programming, which are beyond the scope of this book.

DEALING WITH TIME – DISCOUNTING

Discounting reflects the idea that individuals exhibit 'positive time preference', that is, people prefer to have access to resources and enjoy their use now rather than later. Another way of putting it, is in the axiom that individuals prefer to delay costs for as long as possible and receive benefits as soon as possible. This is summarised in the translation of future costs and benefits into their equivalent net present value (NPV), where the present values of costs and benefits are calculated using the formula:

$$NPV = A/(1 + r)^n$$

Where A is the cost or benefit accrued in year 'n', r is the rate of discount and n is a number equal to or bigger than 0 and serves as an index of time, with the present time being = 0. For example, imagine that the use of alteplase for thrombolysis of patients who have just had AMI is being evaluated. Assuming, for illustrative purposes, that the evidence shows that reduced mortality benefits with alteplase, relative to streptokinase are observed to last for the first 2 years after thrombolysis only. For simplicity, assume that the difference in survival rate between alteplase and streptokinase is constant for those first 2 years and then disappears. Let A (i.e. alteplase use) = 0.01 × 10000=100, that is, 1% of the initial cohort of 10 000 patients would be able to live 2 extra years thanks to the aspirin. Economic theory has been used to argue that the 100 years of life saved in the second year are equivalent in value to $100/(1 + r)$ years saved in the first. In this example using the NPV criterion, total benefits amount to $100 - 100/(1 + r)$, which – because typically $r > 0$ – is lower than 200, the number of years of life saved over the 2-year period.

The reason why discounting health benefits is controversial might seem obvious from the example above: the interpretation of a discounted value for monetary costs is relatively straightforward whereas that of discounting future health benefits does not appear rooted in common sense. From society's perspective, if we believe that health promotion initiatives aimed at improving health in the future (e.g. antismoking programmes) are of value, then a decision to discount future health benefits would severely undermine the value of such programmes in any economic analysis. The annual rate of cost discounting widely used in UK studies is that recommended by the Treasury for publicly financed projects – currently 6% – whereas for benefits NICE's recommendation to manufacturers and sponsors making a submission to a technology appraisal is to discount benefits at an annual rate of 1.5%. This practice contrasts with guidelines adopted in the US, which recommend that both costs and benefits (in QALYs) be discounted at the rate of 3% and that **sensitivity analysis** (see below) varies the rate between 0 and 7%.

The power of discounting is such that any health benefits arising more than 10 years in the future would exert an insignificant impact on the NPV benefit calculation. Equally, on the cost side, we need to address intergenerational issues in healthcare provision – to what extent is it the responsibility of our current generation to invest to meet the healthcare needs of future generations? It is arguable that much of the current stock of hospitals from which we benefit arose as a result of investments made by previous generations. Do we therefore have an obligation to invest in an infrastructure of healthcare for future generations? Again, if the future health benefits arising from such investments are discounted then the value of any such intergenerational effect will be negligible.

DEALING WITH UNCERTAINTY – SENSITIVITY ANALYSIS

Uncertainty might be present in the evaluation for several reasons:

- if data are unavailable and expert opinion is used
- if data are available but are known to be of dubious accuracy
- if there is methodological controversy around the derivation of values.

The vast majority of analyses will be afflicted by one if not all of these sources of uncertainty. In such situations, point estimates are likely to be of limited value in guiding decision making. What the decision maker needs to know is how robust the economic analysis is to 'reasonable' variations in underlying assumptions or parameter values. In cases where a relatively small variation fundamentally alters the conclusions of the analysis then obviously little reliance should be placed upon the results. Alternatively, in cases where the results remain robust (drug A is still preferred to drug B) in the face of 'reasonable' variations in both parameter values and underlying assumptions, then the decision maker can place greater reliance on the accuracy and consistency of the results.

The process of a sensitivity analyses is that the values for important parameters are varied to determine whether the results are sensitive to parameter values or the assumptions made. For example, if efficacy data is used from a cholesterol-lowering drug trial, it is likely that the average risk reduction obtained in the highly controlled trial environment will be used to assess cost effectiveness in an economic evaluation. Given that the effectiveness of the drug in practice is a key parameter, it is likely that this would be varied in a sensitivity analysis. It is widely recognised that the effectiveness of drug therapy in practice is likely to be lower than the efficacy measurements obtained in the tightly controlled environment of a clinical trial. Thus, the efficacy measure could be perceived as being the upper bound of the plausible range of variation for the effect of the drug in practice.

A one-way sensitivity analysis enables the impact of non-compliance and many other real-world elements to be analysed one at a time. Some studies describe their concern with uncertainty relating to the value of key parameters in the model by presenting a 'threshold analysis': the parameter value at which the study results change qualitatively, say, from a new drug having a positive net benefit to having zero net benefits (i.e. equal costs and benefits) is presented separately for variables with the highest uncertainty. In cases of high uncertainty, the practice of substituting the worst possible and most favourable possible values for the uncertain parameter value is recommended. In studies extending beyond a 1-year time frame, a natural choice for sensitivity analysis is the discount rate applied to costs and benefits. The results of the sensitivity analysis can be presented in a table of revised estimates of costs, benefits and ICERs and/or graphically. As a hypothetical example, a CUA study might present its results as a function of the discount rate in terms similar to those in Figure 7.2.

In the case depicted, where only the discounted rate of costs is varied, the ICER when no discounting is applied to future costs is £20 000, whereas as the discount rate is raised to 10% annually the ICER approaches £22 000. Assuming a cost effectiveness threshold of £20 000, the hypothetical therapy considered in this example would be considered good value for money only if it was agreed that costs should not be discounted.

If there is more than one parameter for which uncertainty exists due to lack of or incompleteness of data, then two-way and multiway sensitivity analyses might be more appropriate to assess their importance for the results. Two-way sensitivity analyses create plausible combinations of values for two key parameters with uncertain values and recalculate the results accordingly, and so on for n-way sensitivity analyses, where n is the number of uncertain parameters (e.g. compliance, risk of recrudescence, cost of recrudescence, etc.).

Economic evaluations are often based on data from pragmatic trials reporting statistical measures of precision in the form of confidence intervals

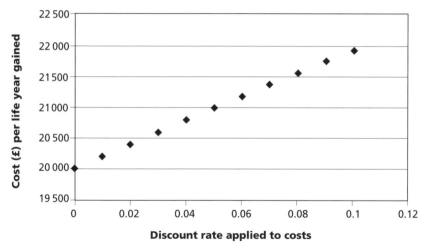

Fig 7.2 The results of a cost utility analysis presented as a function of the discount rate

around the point estimate of effect; the robustness of results to sampling variation in parameter estimates can be assessed using the upper and lower bounds of confidence intervals in sensitivity analysis. Here, sensitivity is used to assess the extent to which results are robust to those extreme values of effectiveness. When there is more than one parameter value with a measure of sample variability attached to it, the ideal type of sensitivity analysis would simulate the range of uncertainty in the results by using some type of probabilistic sampling technique such as that employed in **Monte Carlo** approaches (see Chapter 9).

CONCLUSION

This chapter introduced the principles and practice of pharmacoeconomic evaluation in a non-technical manner. The exposition was based on the principle that pharmacoeconomics contributes to informing the process and rationalising the outcome of healthcare decision making. It does so by systematically presenting the choices faced by the decision maker in terms of expected benefits to achieve and forgo from one, and more often two or more, possible courses of action. Although efficiency considerations are only one of a number of aspects likely to influence decision making (others include equity, affordability, tradition, political pressure, political inertia), their importance is testified by the ongoing development of more advanced methods in pharmacoeconomics and outcomes research and their wider application to drug therapy and public health policy assessment.

REFERENCES

Brown R E, Hutton J, Burrel A 2001 Cost effectiveness of treatment options in advanced breast cancer in the UK. Pharmacoeconomics 19(11):1091–1102

Davey P, Grainger D, MacMillan J et al 1998 Economic evaluation of insulin lispro versus neutral (regular) insulin therapy using a willingness to pay approach. Pharmacoeconomics 13(3):347–358

Dunn C J, Plosker G L 2002 Insulin Lispro. A pharmacoeconomic review of its use in diabetes mellitus. Pharmacoeconomics 20(14):989–1025

Hutton J, Brown R, Borowitz M et al 1996 A new decision model does cost utility comparisons of chemotherapy in recurrent metastatic breast cancer. Pharmacorconomics 9(2):8–22

MacLaine G, Patel H 2001 A cost effectiveness model of alternative statins to achieve target LDL-cholesterol levels. International Journal of Clinical Practice 55(4):243–249

McPherson R, Hanna K, Agro A, Braeken A 2001 Cerivastatin versus branded pravastatin in the treatment of primary hypercholesterolaemia in primary care practice in Canada: a one-year, open label, randomised, comparative study of efficacy, safety, and cost effectiveness. Clinical Therapeutics 23(9):1492–1507

FURTHER READING

Drummond M 1994 Economic analysis alongside controlled trials: an introduction for clinical researchers. Department of Health, London

Drummond M, Stoddard G, Torrance G 1988 Methods for the economic evaluation of healthcare programmes. Oxford Medical Publications, Oxford

Eddy D M 1992 Applying cost effectiveness analysis – the inside story. Journal of the American Medical Association 268(18):2575–2582

Eddy D M 1992 Cost effectiveness analysis – will it be accepted? Journal of the American Medical Association 268(1):132–136

Eddy D M 1992 Cost effectiveness analysis: a conversation with my father. Journal of the American Medical Association 267(12):1669–1675

Eddy D M 1992 Cost effectiveness analysis: is it up to the task? Journal of the American Medical Association 267(24):3342–3348

Hadorn D C 1991 Setting health care priorities in Oregon. Cost effectiveness meets the rule of rescue. Journal of the American Medical Association 265(17):2218–2225

Haycox A, Drummond M, Walley A 1997 Pharmacoeconomics: integrating economic evaluation into clinical trials. British Journal of Clinical Pharmacology 43:559–562

Jefferson T, Demicheli V, Mugford M 1996 Elementary economic evaluation in health care. BMJ Publishing Group, London

Johannesson M, Weinstein M 1996 Designing and conducting cost–benefit analyses. In: Spilker B, ed. Quality of life and pharmacoeconomics in clinical trials, 2nd edn. Lippincott–Raven, Philadelphia, p 1085–1092

Normand C 1991 Economics, health and the economics of health. British Medical Journal 303:1572–1577

Robinson R 1993 Economic evaluation and health care: cost benefit analysis. British Medical Journal 307:924–926

Robinson R 1993 Costs and cost minimisation analysis. British Medical Journal 307:726–728

Robinson R 1993 Economic evaluation and health care: cost effectiveness analysis. British Medical Journal 307:793–795

Robinson R 1993 Economic evaluation and health care: cost utility analysis. British Medical Journal 307:859–862

Robinson R 1993 What does it mean? British Medical Journal 307:670–673

Viney R, Lancsar E, Louviere J 2002 Discrete choice experiments to measure consumer preferences for health and healthcare. Expert Review of Pharamcoeconomics and Outcomes Research 2(4):319–326

Walley T, Haycox A 1997 Pharmacoeconomics: basic concepts and terminology. British Journal of Clinical Pharmacology 43(4):343–347

Pharmacoeconomics and clinical trials

8

INTRODUCTION

The information needs of health services have altered fundamentally; although clinical trials are the best source of early clinical information, these evaluations are now generally perceived as incomplete. It is no longer sufficient for pharmaceutical companies to generate data on safety and **efficacy**. Throughout the world, regulators and payers increasingly require information on cost effectiveness to enable them to make more informed decisions about the value for money provided by new drugs. In this changing environment, pharmaceutical companies must alter and enhance their clinical trial programmes to generate economic as well as clinical information that could be used to inform pharmacoeconomic analyses.

Clinical trials are currently designed to achieve two main objectives:

- to assess the safety of new drugs
- to assess the efficacy of new drugs.

These, together with the need to achieve a minimum level of quality in the production process are the three 'hurdles' that a drug currently has to surmount to obtain marketing approval from national regulatory authorities. However, the increasing need to prove 'value for money' at the time of product launch has led to attempts to investigate the cost effectiveness of new drugs within the context of clinical trials. Previously, most pharmacoeconomic analyses were conducted in conjunction with Phase IV clinical trials as part of the postmarketing surveillance process, which enabled them to assess cost effectiveness in real-world clinical practice. The increased emphasis on premarketing clinical-trial-based economic evaluation reflects a growing recognition that decision makers need evidence of cost effectiveness at an early stage in the life cycle of a drug.

Economic evaluations place additional pressures on both researchers and patients in clinical studies by adding to the outcome variables to be measured. Information must be generated on factors such as resource use and quality of life, as well as on the clinical end-points.

A clinical trial is an intensive data-gathering episode with a crowded agenda, even when it is restricted to analysing drug safety and efficacy. Adding on the requirement to assess cost effectiveness risks adversely affecting the evaluation of safety and efficacy. How, then, can pharmacoeconomic information be

Concept box 8.1 – Linking efficacy to effectiveness

There are many reasons why a drug that proves efficacious in clinical trials might have a reduced therapeutic effect in mainstream clinical practice. Patients in such trials can be highly selected, both to exclude more 'difficult' patients and to emphasise patients who are more likely to comply with therapy. Such selectivity is obviously not possible in mainstream clinical practice. The greatest dilutory impact, however, is likely to be related to lower levels of compliance in mainstream clinical practice. During a trial, a patient's drug use is closely monitored ensuring that non-compliance is minimised. In real-world clinical practice, the absence of such close surveillance is likely to lead to a significant level of non-compliance with drug therapy. The 'forgiveness' exhibited by individual drugs (how well their therapeutic effect is maintained in the face of non-compliance) will be a major determinant of how successfully the results obtained in clinical trials can be translated to actual clinical practice.

generated without diverting attention and resources away from the overriding clinical objectives of a trial?

A clinical trial designed to evaluate drug efficacy and safety is not an ideal environment in which to assess the comparative cost effectiveness of any new drug. Although such trials provide invaluable clinical data on the efficacy of an intervention, and thus exhibit high internal validity, they generalise poorly as proxies for the cost effectiveness of interventions in normal clinical practice and thus exhibit low external validity. As well as possible bias in the trial (e.g. choice of a suboptimal dosage for the comparator drug), many further opportunities for bias occur when integrating pharmacoeconomic analyses into clinical trials. Opportunities for bias include the choice of economic technique (inappropriately using **cost minimisation analysis** (CMA) when the drugs being compared have different outcomes), **perspective** (the choice of a limited perspective when important costs are imposed elsewhere) and methodological assumptions (informing an **economic model** with a biased or partial review of the evidence base). In the latter case, bias will be far less visible because it can be hidden within the assumptions underlying the analysis rather than in the information base or structure of the analysis itself.

The clinical trial process therefore provides a unique opportunity to generate valuable pharmacoeconomic information that can be made available to health-care decision makers at the time of product launch. Unfortunately, the very controlled nature of the clinical trial process (its main value in addressing clinical issues) provides problems in interpreting the pharmacoeconomic data derived from this source. The conundrum facing pharmacoeconomic research is how to translate the credible and scientific data obtained within the clinical trial framework to predict the cost effectiveness of a drug in mainstream clinical practice.

One of the major implications of incorporating pharmacoeconomic data relates to the need to identify, measure and value resource utilisation within the clinical trials framework. The 'boundaries' of the cost analysis depend upon the perspective from which the trial is being undertaken. The narrowest perspective simply requires the direct costs (all costs arising as a direct consequence of use of the new drug) to be assessed. A broader analysis would incorporate an evaluation of **indirect costs**, which value the impact of changes in health status and productivity into the cost analysis. The widest definition of costs incorporates the concept of 'intangible' costs and would require the analysis to place a cost on factors such as the pain being experienced by patients treated in the clinical trial.

THE INTERPRETATION OF PHARMACOECONOMIC ANALYSES BASED ON CLINICAL TRIALS

For both clinicians and health service policy makers, perhaps the greatest difficulties lie in interpreting what degree of reliability should be placed on pharmacoeconomic analyses attached to clinical trials. Such evaluations should be scientifically based, timely and focused on addressing the information needs of healthcare decision makers. Such factors are crucially dependent on the extent to which the results obtained in the trial are generalisable and hence have relevance to mainstream clinical practice. Such generalisability must be assessed carefully.

Clinical trials are based on the concept of hypothesis testing. In addressing the chosen hypothesis, confidence intervals are calculated that provide assurance to a predetermined statistical probability that the true population parameter for a certain variable is contained within a certain statistical range. The technique of choice for dealing with uncertainty related to pharmacoeconomic data is use of **cost effectiveness acceptability curves** (see Chapter 9).

Bayesian analysis is increasingly used in pharmacoeconomic analyses and differs markedly from the approach normally employed in clinical trials. The Bayesian approach is to delineate a probability distribution for the variable of interest in the trial based on a predetermined probability distribution derived from data collected prior to the trial. Generating such prior knowledge requires existing information or the use of a pilot study to obtain information on probability distribution before undertaking the full clinical trial. The analyst continues to compare this prior probability distribution with data generated from the clinical trial to assess the extent to which such prior expectations are supported by results obtained within the clinical trial.

Pharmacoeconomic analyses can be deterministic or stochastic in nature. Deterministic analyses analyse costs and effects as point estimates on the basis that data are largely derived from secondary sources and therefore lack sampling variations. In such analyses the impact of uncertainty is normally explored through the extensive use of **sensitivity analysis**. However, in the case where pharmacoeconomic analyses are integrated into clinical trials, the results should be presented in a stochastic fashion (a mean with an associated variance) with the reliability that should be placed on the results being captured by the confidence intervals surrounding the means. In interpreting the results of such studies, it is important to consider the nature of the distribution of resource use and cost data, which might be highly skewed, especially if a small proportion of patients consumes a large proportion of total resources. For example, when analysing the cost effectiveness of immunisation:

- a small number of patients might suffer severe side-effects that result in hospitalisation and even death
- the majority of patients receive no benefit because, even in the absence of immunisation, they would not have contracted the disease against which they are being protected
- a small proportion who would have contracted the disease in the absence of immunisation receive a great benefit as a consequence of avoiding an extended (and costly) period of hospitalisation or even death.

Given such a distribution of costs and benefits, it becomes obvious that we are not dealing with normal distributions of patient resource use. Both log transformations of skewed data and non-parametric tests can be used to analyse skewed economic data.

The complementary use of confidence interval and sensitivity analyses is therefore important in identifying the reliability of results of pharmacoeconomic analyses. However, in choosing the appropriate approach it is important to recognise that confidence intervals are only appropriate for samples taken from a normal distribution and generate misleading results in situations where the distribution underlying the sample is skewed.

THE TIMING OF PHARMACOECONOMIC EVALUATION

Pharmacoeconomic analyses should be integrated into clinical trials at each stage of the drug-development process. The nature and focus of early analyses, however, are largely aimed at assisting those within the pharmaceutical industry charged with the stop-go decision with regard to further drug development. Pharmacoeconomic evaluation at this very early stage of the process is therefore largely targeted on the internal decision-making process of identifying potentially valuable gaps in the marketplace that would reward further development of the drug by the pharmaceutical company. The majority of new chemical entities (NCEs) developed to this stage are likely to be discontinued for safety or scientific reasons, making it unwise for either the pharmaceutical industry or industry regulators to undertake detailed economic evaluations until the future development of the NCE appears more secure. The cost of such 'wasted' effort, however, has to be balanced by the value of obtaining earlier knowledge of potential market opportunities. The value of earlier information for health professionals primarily relates to their ability to set aside resources and plan to manage the introduction of new drugs. For example, in the UK, the National Institute for Clinical Excellence (NICE) has explicitly recognised the value of early information through the development of its 'horizon scanning' unit, whose aim is to identify – at an early stage in their development – drugs that are likely to impose significant resource implications on the NHS. As the process of drug development continues, however, the principal 'audience' for pharmacoeconomic information increasingly shifts from the pharmaceutical industry to healthcare regulators. The principal audience for economic data obtained in Phase III trials is government agencies charged with controlling, targeting and **reimbursement** of new drugs (e.g. NICE in the UK) and commissioners and providers of healthcare who directly manage the introduction and funding of any new drug.

Concept box 8.3 – Aims of horizon scanning

To identify new and emerging health techniques that might require urgent evaluation, consideration of clinical and cost impact or modification of clinical guidance.

Once the drug has progressed beyond its earliest stages of development, Phase II trials can provide data to identify in greater detail the costs and benefits that are likely to arise from the drug under development. Phase II trials provide the perfect opportunity to fine-tune sample size calculations in readiness for Phase III trials and the ability to pilot proposed documentation such as case report forms and clinical and economic evaluation measures. In addition, early economic models can be developed, tested and refined using Phase II trial data to structure and inform more advanced models for use in Phase III trials. By the end of Phase II, decisions on economic end-points, structures of economic analysis and timeframe for economic analysis should be in place before proceeding to Phase III clinical and economic analyses. Phase II data can also be used to define the most important resource costs to be collected in Phase III, and to provide initial indications as to their likely distribution (Schulman et al 1996).

Postmarketing economic analyses (Phase IV) allow the cost effectiveness of new drugs in clinical practice to be assessed. However, this benefit has to be balanced by the importance of undertaking economic evaluations at an earlier (i.e. premarketing) stage in the life cycle of a product. Any economic analysis based on earlier trials should be further evaluated in a Phase IV real-world clinical practice environment. This will assess any disparity in the estimates of cost effectiveness of drugs in the pre- and postmarketing stages.

INTEGRATING ECONOMIC ANALYSIS INTO CLINICAL TRIALS

Phase III trials are the major source of prelicensing economic data on cost efficacy. Pharmacoeconomic evaluations can be incorporated into Phase III clinical trials in a number of ways:

- a clinical trial can be undertaken specifically to generate data to inform the pharmacoeconomic evaluation
- more frequently, a pharmacoeconomic evaluation can be undertaken as a secondary objective within a clinical trial whose primary aim is to address a clinical hypothesis
- pharmacoeconomic modelling can be used retrospectively to analyse data generated in the clinical trial.

Clinical trials are of comparatively short duration and modelling techniques can be used to extrapolate trial results to identify the long-term costs and benefits that would be likely in clinical practice. Particularly in the case of chronic diseases, clinical trials can provide very limited evidence of how the treatment evaluated will affect the long-term costs of supporting patients and the future health experience of patients. For example, within the comparatively short-term timeframe of a clinical trial, renal transplantation might appear to be an expensive treatment option in comparison to renal dialysis. However, when a pharmacoeconomic model is used to analyse long-term costs and benefits arising from the alternative treatments available, the lifetime resource savings and quality of life improvements associated with transplantation would, for the majority of patients, appear to make this a highly cost-effective long-term intervention.

A further problem encountered when integrating pharmacoeconomic analysis into clinical trials relates to the comparator employed. Head-to-head comparisons between alternative treatment options enable clinicians to compare their performance in a single trial with common outcome measures, inclusion criteria and timeframes of analysis. Placebo-controlled trials are of limited value because they enable indirect comparisons to be made between drugs evaluated in trials that may exhibit significantly different patient populations, outcome measures and timeframes.

In addition, it is important to ensure that the apparent incremental **effectiveness** of a new drug is not being boosted artificially by an inappropriate comparison with an old generation drug (possibly used at suboptimal doses) that is no longer prescribed to any significant extent by clinicians. Ideally, the comparator used in pharmacoeconomic studies should be the current '**gold standard**' treatment of choice, which enables clinicians to compare new treatments directly with their existing therapeutic preference.

PHARMACOECONOMIC DATA COLLECTION – THE PRACTICALITIES

As previously emphasised, economic data collection differs markedly from that normally encountered in clinical trials and care is required to ensure that the demands of economic data collection can be incorporated seamlessly into the clinical trial framework. To achieve this, it is necessary for health economists, clinicians and clinical scientists to collaborate closely in the development of both clinical and economic protocols. The economic component needs to be seen as a vital part of the overall study design and staff should be trained to undertake the economic data collection in a high-quality manner.

Given the importance of pharmacoeconomic evaluations to decision makers, there are growing demands on clinical research personnel to be involved in the integration of pharmacoeconomic studies into the clinical trial framework. Whereas specialist health economists might be required to design and analyse the results of such trials, the responsibility for data extraction inevitably falls upon non-specialists. For this reason, it is important for clinical researchers to enhance their understanding of **pharmacoeconomics** and develop their skills in this area.

The nature of the treatment 'outcomes' used in economic evaluations is likely to be unfamiliar to clinical scientists. Although patient survival obviously remains a key outcome measure, pharmacoeconomic analyses supplement such data by what perhaps could be interpreted as 'softer' outcome measures, such as quality of life and patient satisfaction. Outcome data can be collected directly from individual patients within the trial through interviews, quality-of-life questionnaires or by assessing patient preferences. These are likely to be outside the range of measures normally included in a clinical trial. Obviously, wherever possible, it is desirable to collect resource and quality-of-life data on all of the patients included in the clinical trial. However, where resource constraints make this impossible, detailed and robust resource and quality-of-life information can be collected on an appropriately selected 10% or 20% sample of the study subjects. In certain cases, however, ethical or practical constraints might make it impossible to collect data directly from patients within the trial. It might be necessary to run a parallel exercise to collect data either from patients outside the trial or from historical practice. To 'marry up' the two data sets, however, researchers will have to justify the appropriateness of the results gained outside the trial to the patient group in the clinical study.

Clinicians, clinical scientists and health economists must agree on the feasibility and importance of the economic component of the trial prior to study initiation. In addition, full details of the data requirements of the economic protocol must be provided and explained fully to study participants.

A number of necessary prerequisites have been identified that must be completed before initiating economic data collection (Mauskopf et al 1996):

- The first requirement is to develop a comprehensive economic plan that addresses issues such as study design, research hypothesis, choice of comparators, choice of methodology, choice of data collection instruments and primary and secondary end-points.
- The next requirement is to design a data collection strategy, the case report form (CRF) and prepare written guidelines for CRF completion.
- Investigator training is then required, together with design of a database, development of a source documentation verification plan and design of patient consent forms.
- Log sheets must then be developed to record the completeness of patients' self-report data.
- The economic plan must be fully developed and validated before the CRFs are designed to ensure that all required data is collected but that no excess data items are collected for which no analysis is planned.

Close collaboration and extensive communication between all personnel involved is crucial to the successful implementation of a combined clinical and economic trial. Mauskopf et al (1996) also identified necessary activities required to be undertaken during the clinical trial. These include:

- review of CRFs and log sheets
- verification of source documentation
- ensuring adequate data collection
- readjustment of protocol or CRF as required.

Preparation of an investigator newsletter is also encouraged to enhance communication between investigators. Once all the necessary data has been collected, it becomes necessary to implement the agreed economic analysis plan, which outlines the structure and nature of the economic analysis to be undertaken.

Clinical trials, by their very nature, extrapolate away from real-world clinical practice. Clinical trials require increased monitoring of patients and facilitate strict selection of patients, which artificially alters both the costs and benefits derived within the trial. The nature of the trial is likely to increase the level of healthcare resources consumed by patients and, to generalise trial costs to mainstream clinical practice, such **protocol-driven costs** must be excluded from the analysis. Similarly, the clinical benefits identified in the trial must be evaluated to assess their generalisability to mainstream clinical practice.

Such protocol-driven costs and benefits are a source of potential bias in all RCT-based economic evaluations because they can artificially alter the apparent cost effectiveness of the treatment options being evaluated. For example, as part of its protocol, a clinical trial of a proton pump inhibitor might require all patients to undergo routine endoscopy to assess the clinical improvement resulting from treatment. To extrapolate away from protocol-driven to real-world costs, it is necessary to determine what proportion of patients treated with proton pump inhibitors in a real-world clinical setting

> **Concept box 8.4 – Protocol-driven costs**
>
> Just as the efficacy measured in clinical trials can vary from effectiveness in clinical practice, costs measured in trials can vary from costs that are likely to arise in mainstream clinical practice. Certain diagnostic tests/investigations might be required to assess the efficacy of therapy and hence to evaluate outcome. In mainstream clinical practice, such tests/investigations would be used less frequently because their use would be driven by clinical considerations (the symptoms exhibited by the individual patient) rather than protocol requirements. To assess the expected resource impact of therapy in mainstream clinical practice, it is necessary to identify and extract such protocol-driven costs from consideration.

would be likely to have a clinically driven need for such a diagnostic procedure.

Within protocol-driven costs, it is perhaps helpful to distinguish between 'protocol-prescribed' and 'protocol-derived' costs:

Protocol-prescribed costs. These refer to resource use required by patients as part of the clinical trial protocol. Patients might require frequent clinical visits to assess changes in surrogate outcomes and adverse event monitoring, which could falsely increase resource use above that required in clinical practice. In addition, the rigid treatment regimen required in clinical trials might restrict clinical freedom to reduce treatment intensity if a patient's condition were to improve, thus failing to reflect improvements in resource use that might occur in mainstream clinical practice.

Protocol-derived costs. By contrast, these occur when the trial process leads to the identification and treatment of disease that might not have been identified otherwise. The enhanced clinical diagnosis and surveillance exhibited in a clinical trial might, therefore, identify health problems that require additional treatment. A distinction must therefore be made between resource use that is related to the clinical trial design and the level of resource use required for strictly clinical purposes. To achieve this, analysts must be aware not just of the level of resource use but also of the reasons for such resource use within the clinical trial environment. This can be achieved through direct observation of clinical practice, use of large-scale medical databases or by resorting to expert opinion.

ECONOMICS, CLINICAL TRIALS AND SAMPLE SIZE CALCULATIONS

A major problem facing RCT-based economic evaluations is the estimation of a sample size that is adequate to identify statistically significant differences in resource use between the different arms of the trial. Frequently, sample sizes that are sufficient to identify statistically significant differences in clinical variables are inadequate to achieve statistical significance in economic variables. A range of potential solutions has been suggested to overcome this problem. The use of a predetermined 'threshold' value of cost effectiveness that determines the point at which an acceptable level of cost effectiveness is achieved would enable power calculations to be undertaken for economic analyses. Prior knowledge of confidence intervals would therefore be helpful in determining appropriate sample sizes for economic analyses.

Powering a clinical trial specifically to address cost effectiveness also raises a range of practical and ethical issues. The range of end-points considered in an economic evaluation tends to be far broader than the clinical end-points assessed. Economic variables also tend to have a broader variability, requiring greater sample sizes to achieve statistical significance. It is unlikely that any ethical committee would sanction the extension of a clinical trial beyond the point at which clinical superiority might be statistically proven. However, even in cases where clinical trials can be powered on economic variables, ethical problems can arise in submitting patients to trial risk simply to evaluate the existence of economically important differences. There is, therefore, likely to be no practical alternative to powering trials on the basis of clinical differences while using sensitivity analysis to evaluate the robustness of the economic analysis. So when incorporating pharmacoeconomic analyses into a clinical trial, it is not normal to alter the sample size to accommodate the economic analysis but, as in the clinical trial, the greater the number of patients evaluated the more useful the results are likely to be. However, it is also important to recognise that as the number of patients included in a clinical trial increases so too does the cost of the trial.

Concept box 8.5 – Sample sizes and power calculations in pharmacoeconomics

Undertaking a power calculation for pharmacoeconomic analyses is complicated by the number of individual resources (inpatient admissions, GP attendances, drug costs, diagnostic tests, etc.) that need to be combined to estimate the cost of treatment during the period of the trial. Such estimates are also complicated by significant cost variations occurring between individual patients, with the most expensive resources (inpatient stays) frequently being comparatively rare and highly variable. Cost estimates, therefore, would require larger sample sizes to achieve comparative discriminatory power to clinical analyses. The ethical basis for extending a trial to pursue economic end-points once a definitive clinical outcome has been reached is open to question. In such circumstances, the normal approach is to accept the sample size indicated to effectively address the clinical hypothesis and to make extensive use of sensitivity analysis to address remaining levels of uncertainty in the pharmacoeconomic analysis.

A typical RCT will have one or two primary clinical end-points and the sample size for the trial will be based on well-established clinical event rates in current practice. By contrast, economic trials must evaluate variations in the use of numerous health resources that together determine the estimated cost of treatment throughout the period of the study. To obtain such a variety of information, it is often necessary to collect patient-based information from a wide range of sources (e.g. inpatient data, outpatient data, hospital pharmacies, hospital laboratories, ambulance services and GPs). This data collection procedure is resource intensive and the overall quality of the analysis depends on the least reliable of the many sources employed. This is of enhanced importance given that, in many analyses, the least frequent resource-consuming events (e.g. inpatient stays) might also be the most expensive. This is a key point and means that cost estimates are likely to suffer from a higher degree of uncertainty than efficacy estimates. Given the additional variability attached to cost estimation in pharmacoeconomic trials, such studies would generally require greater patient numbers to achieve comparable discriminatory power to clinical trials. Powering a trial for cost effectiveness would be likely to substantially increase the number of cases required over a trial powered for clinical end-points alone. Perhaps therefore it is not surprising that the normal approach is to power clinical trials on the basis of clinical end-points, with the pharmacoeconomic analysis passively accepting the size of trial determined by clinical criteria and dealing with uncertainty through sensitivity analysis.

When designing a pharmacoeconomic study, detailed pretrial costing studies can optimise the value of economic data from clinical trials by evaluating the relative significance of individual elements within the overall cost estimate. This enables the economic analysis to focus within the trial on individual resources that are the most significant determinants of overall care costs. If it is accepted that pharmacoeconomic analyses cannot achieve the levels of statistical significance achieved for clinical variables, then one corollary might be the need to accept lower evidential criteria or, alternatively, to adopt an entirely different basis of assessment for economic analyses based on clinical trials.

CLINICAL TRIALS AND ECONOMIC MODELLING

Efficacy is frequently measured in clinical trials using short-term indicators that might not capture all the long-term effects of a particular intervention. The use of such time-limited end-points makes it difficult to evaluate the impact of drugs on long-term health outcomes. Thus, to assess the true long-term value of drugs, we need to develop methods to extrapolate data collected from clinical trials into the future. This is an aim of economic modelling.

An economic model tries to model the real-world costs and benefits arising from different therapeutic strategies. It is a data-hungry procedure because all significant therapeutic pathways (together with their associated transitional probabilities and resultant costs and benefits) must be incorporated into the model. Inevitably, the analysis will encounter many areas in which 'evidence' is either completely unavailable or has been generated outside a controlled clinical trial. The breadth of information needed for an economic model will require the application of 'evidence' from sources of varying quality, including 'expert opinion' if objective empirical data are currently unavailable. The model and economic evaluation should be continually updated if new and relevant clinical and/or economic data become available. Models require each stage of a comprehensive decision tree to be informed by the best available data from sources such as systematic reviews of the available clinical evidence. Unfortunately, such high-quality sources are only rarely available and the choice of data source is frequently pragmatic. The robustness of such models needs to be interpreted in relation to the quality of their underlying data and assumptions. Therefore, the source and nature of such assumptions and data sources must be made as transparent as possible. The potential benefits derived from economic modelling are described more fully in Chapter 9.

The value of incorporating economic analyses into clinical trials is only partly related to the ability to derive a definitive economic conclusion based on the results of a single (possibly atypical) trial. These analyses also enable health economists to identify the patterns of resource use which represents the essential building blocks for pharmacoeconomic modelling. The information obtained from trials and modelling is mutually supportive because it addresses different but complementary issues. However, this different focus means that modelling cannot be supplanted by larger and longer RCTs because although these would provide more evidence to be incorporated into the modelling process, for reasons of ethics and cost they are unlikely ever to be carried out.

Economic modelling still suffers from a general perception among clinical scientists that it is simply a poor substitute for trial-based analysis. By contrast, Langley (1997) emphasises the superiority of modelling over clinical trials in evaluating real-world cost effectiveness given the difficulty in generalising the results of trial-based economic evaluations to real-life clinical practice. Economic modelling also allows clinicians to adapt the results obtained in clinical trials to local cost structures and local clinical practice. Clinical trials provide little evidence concerning the extent to which clinical benefits can be replicated in the real world. The robustness of clinical trial results can be assessed only when the drug has been used in clinical practice for some time. In addition, cost effectiveness in clinical practice will be continuously improving as the prescriber's experience with the new drug increases.

Concept box 8.6 – Using clinical trials and economic modelling

1. Can predict and compare expected health outcomes of interventions under uncertain conditions
2. Can compare the risk-adjusted costs of competing interventions
3. Helps to inform decision-making in a systematic manner.

PHARMACOECONOMICS AND MULTINATIONAL CLINICAL TRIALS

Fundamental differences exist in the ability to transfer economic data and clinical data across national boundaries. The clinical data (e.g. changes in blood pressure or cholesterol levels in response to drug treatment) are likely to be largely consistent between the populations of different countries so that clinical results can largely be extrapolated across national boundaries. By contrast, economic data is not an objective variable but rather an artefact generated by summing a wide range of resources weighted by a structure of unit costs that varies widely between countries. As a consequence, cost effectiveness analyses undertaken in one country are unlikely to be directly applicable in others, and might even be of limited applicability in different locations within the country of analysis. In this respect, pharmacoeconomic analyses generate results that are largely time and location specific, and multinational studies therefore provide particular challenges in the generation and interpretation of economic data. The structure of costs and methods of clinical practice are likely to vary significantly between each country of analysis because of differences in the structure of health services, local prices or local medical practice. For example, there is little to indicate that the clinical impact resulting from use of a proton pump inhibitor would vary significantly between patients from different countries. However, the cost effectiveness of the proton pump inhibitor will be determined by nationally specific factors such as comparative drug prices and differences in local medical practice (who prescribes it, to which patients, at what stage in the disease process and with what associated pathway of care). All of which leads to significant variations in measured cost effectiveness derived in different healthcare systems. In addition, any attempt to derive an 'average' of each country's cost effectiveness ratios would lead to a meaningless cost effectiveness ratio of relevance to no particular individual country.

Local units costs and medical practice will vary widely between individual countries, with diagnostic procedures and treatments that are used widely in one country being used rarely in other countries. Variations in the structure of health-service provision might also reduce the applicability of the treatment results between countries. For example, the UK has a well-developed structure of primary care health services that determine the cost and nature of a 'primary care consultation'. However, a similar consultation in a country in which such an initial clinical consultation is more intensive (with the patient spending a longer time with the clinician and having a wider range of diagnostic tests) would incur a higher unit cost.

In addition to such structural variability a range of operational differences might make it difficult to generalise cost effectiveness results across national boundaries. For example, the market share of different drugs used to treat a particular disease might vary widely between different countries; drug utilisation is also likely to vary between individual countries. Estimates concerning the weighted **average cost** of each category of drug used will depend on the national market share of each individual drug, and this is likely to vary enormously between each of the countries analysed. Similarly, the comparative availability and utilisation of different diagnostic tests will also vary widely between different countries. It is therefore easy to perceive the difficulties of generalising the results of cost effectiveness analyses across national boundaries.

CONCLUSIONS

Given the increasing proportion of healthcare resources devoted to the drugs bill in all countries, questions relating to the introduction and targeting of a new drug are inevitably both clinical and economic in nature. It is now more readily accepted, therefore, that clinical trials should not be undertaken without consideration of the wider economic implications of treatment and the logic for integrating economic analyses into traditional clinical trials is compelling. As this chapter has argued, however, resource and quality-of-life data captured in a clinical trial need to be interpreted with extreme caution in extrapolating towards real-world clinical practice. There is no 'gold standard' for such trial design, unlike the RCT utilised in clinical analysis. As this chapter has emphasised, the applicability and interpretation of clinical and economic data is different and it is vital for clinical scientists to be aware of such differences.

Clinical trials evaluate the efficacy of therapy in the hands of specialists in an environment of clinical certainty. By contrast, economic models focus on evaluating the effectiveness of therapy in a real-world clinical environment characterised by clinical uncertainty, and in which therapy is prescribed and consumed under less then ideal conditions.

The economic focus on effectiveness, therefore, implicitly incorporates the impact of real-world clinical issues, such as non-compliance and suboptimal drug utilisation, which are, for good reason, controlled in the context of a clinical trial. The extrapolation from trials to real-world clinical practice can be achieved through the use of medical databases or direct observation to identify costs and benefits that arise in clinical practice but are artificially controlled by the research protocol. In this manner, pharmacoeconomic models must specifically incorporate the large number of confounding variables that interfere with the 'pure' relationship between drug use and patient response isolated in clinical trials.

REFERENCES

Langley P C 1997 The future of pharmacoeconomics: a commentary. Clinical Therapeutics 19(4):762–769
Mauskopf J, Schulman K, Bell L, Glick H 1996 A strategy for collecting pharmacoeconomic data during phase II/III trials. Pharmacoeconomics 3:264–277
Schulman K A, Llana T, Yabroff K R 1996 Economic assessment within the clinical development programme. Medical Care 34(12):89–95

Pharmacoeconomics and clinical trials

Modelling in health economics

9

INTRODUCTION

Although we are not aware of it, every day we reap the benefits of computer models and simulations. Chances are, the cars we drive were at least partly developed based on computer simulations – everything from the engine to the aerodynamics and the assembly line used to build it. Every morning, the weather forecast represents the culmination of hours of computing time, generating simulations from complex models of weather patterns populated with data collected from weather stations. Similarly, health economists use computer models to generate cost effectiveness estimates to predict how efficient a healthcare intervention is. This chapter describes the principles of modelling in **pharmacoeconomics** and, using illustratory examples, aims to help the reader to gain an understanding of the methods used.

MODELS IN HEALTH ECONOMICS

Models can be thought of as simplifications of the real world, where the essence of reality is captured but, in accordance with Occam's razor, much of the complicating excess baggage that accompanies reality is dispensed (see Concept box 9.1). When using models to assist clinical decision making in pharmacoeconomics, the more important aspects that need to be accounted for can include the **effectiveness** and adverse effects associated with each competing medicine, treatment costs and the costs associated with treatment failure and side-effects. What might be considered as 'excess baggage' can include consequences that might occur with very low probability or that are associated with low adverse health risk, and costs that are minimal compared to other 'cost drivers'. To include these in the model will merely complicate the analysis without adding great value. Models aim to simplify the issues relevant to decision making while avoiding the problems of inaccuracy (which might be evident if the model were too simple).

In health economic evaluation, models are typically used to decide between two or more treatment pathways if the relevant clinical trials have not been conducted or are impossible for ethical or logistical reasons, or if they were not designed to capture economic data. The decision of which pathway is

Concept box 9.2 – Decision analysis

Decision analysis is a prescriptive way of analysing problems or decisions, allowing for clinical and economic consequences of medical actions, and for attitudes, to be analysed under conditions of uncertainty. The probability and consequence of each possible event are stated explicitly. Decision analyses are frequently depicted as decision trees where decisions are represented as squares (decision nodes) and circles denote chance nodes, where future events are beyond the control of the decision maker and the outcome is uncertain. Branches represent different treatment options (when they originate from decision nodes) or different treatment consequences (when they originate from chance nodes).

optimal will depend on how effective (and free from adverse effects) and how expensive each option is. The treatments available will be associated with many uncertainties – indeed, the practice of medicine is inherently very uncertain: What is the effectiveness of drug A? What are the chances it will produce an undesired side-effect? What are the alternative treatments and how effective are they? – the list is potentially endless. **Decision analysis** is a systematic approach to decision making under such conditions of uncertainty. It is: (i) explicit, (ii) quantitative and (iii) prescriptive in that it:

- makes the analyst structure the decision problem in a framework that captures the key elements of the process under evaluation
- requires each decision and consequence relating to the choice made to be valued in terms of probability, cost and outcome
- is intended to help physicians and other healthcare decision makers decide what they should do under a given set of circumstances.

Decision analytic models are often depicted as 'decision trees' (Fig. 9.1). In the example that follows, the currently available drug, A, is compared with a more expensive but more effective drug, B. This model is available electronically at www.liv.ac.uk/prg/model.xls. The decision is whether to introduce drug B as first-line therapy or to reserve its use for patients in whom drug A has failed. By convention, decisions within decision trees are represented by square

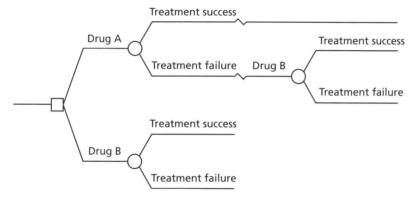

Fig 9.1 A decision tree representing the treatment options for hypothetical drugs A and B

Table 9.1   Parameter estimates for the costs and probabilities used in the decision tree illustrated in Fig. 9.1

Parameter	Deterministic	Stochastic
Effectiveness of A (p)	0.6	Beta (21,14)
Effectiveness of B (q)	0.9	Beta (80,9)
Effectiveness of B (r) after failure with A	0.5	Beta (20,20)
Cost of successful treatment with A	£1500	
Cost of unsuccessful treatment with A	£200	Log normal (5.3,0.1)
Cost of successful treatment with B	£2000	
Cost of unsuccessful treatment with B	£500	Log normal (6.2,1)
Cost of unsuccessful treatment with B after failing with A	£1000	Log normal (6.6,1)
Cost of successful treatment with B after failing with A	£750	Log normal (6.9,1)
Utility associated with treatment success	0.8	Beta (12,3)
Utility associated with treatment failure	0.6	Beta (140,93)

decision nodes. The chances (probability) of treatment success, p for treatment A and q for treatment B, are complimented by the probability of treatment failure $(1 - p)$ and $(1 - q)$, respectively (Table 9.1). A third probability, r, represents the chances of treatment success with drug B in cases where A has previously failed. We might expect r to be less than q because only treatment failures (to A) are selected. Typically, estimates for parameters p, q and r are obtained from clinical trials. Chance nodes are, by convention, denoted as circles.

In addition to including the effectiveness of the treatment, we also have to incorporate the costs and outcomes associated with each treatment pathway. For example, if a patient is successfully treated with drug A, a cost of £1500 will be incurred. The **utility** score associated with the health state of being successfully treated is 0.8 (Table 9.1, first and second columns). These values are point estimates, representing the average effect or cost of a drug in a trial, and form the basis of a deterministic model – one that does not take into account uncertainty in the parameter estimates (Fig. 9.2).

The process of determining the expected costs and benefits associated with a stepped approach first-line therapy, given the probabilities of treatment success or failure, is often referred to as 'rolling back'. The process is as follows:

For patients treated with drug B as first-line therapy:

Expected costs are (£2000 × 0.9) + (£500 × 0.1) = £1850
Expected benefits are (0.8 × 0.9) + (0.6 × 0.1) = 0.78 utilities

For patients subjected to a stepped care approach (A then B):

Expected costs is the sum of: 0.6 × {£1500} + 0.4 × {0.5 × (£1000 + £200) + 0.5 × (£200 + £750)} = £1330
Expected benefits is the sum of: 0.6 × {0.8} + 0.4 × {0.5 × 0.8 + 0.5 × 0.6} = 0.76 utilities

On average, therefore, the expected costs and benefits of treating patients with drug B as first-line therapy are higher than a stepped care approach. Given these figures, the incremental cost effectiveness ratio (ICER) is as follows:

$$\text{ICER} = \frac{£1850 - £1330}{0.78 - 0.76} = £26\,000 \text{ per QALY gained}$$

The attractiveness of modelling is the flexibility that it offers to the user:

1. It allows data from numerous sources to be combined (Nuijten 1998). In the simple example given here, treatment effectiveness could have been derived from clinical trials or from a meta-analysis of trials; cost data from local or national sources and utilities from trials or surveys. It is unlikely, particularly when more complex models comparing numerous alternatives are considered, that all the data can be obtained from a single study.

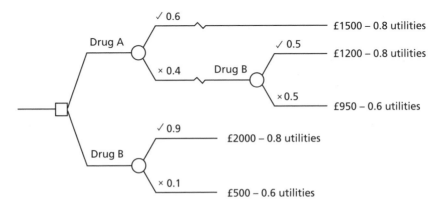

Fig 9.2 A decision tree representing the treatment options for hypothetical drugs A and B, also indicating the probabilities of treatment success (✔) and failure (✗), costs and outcomes

2. Given that parameter estimates might be changed, e.g. costs or disease **prevalence**, cost effectiveness estimates can be generated that reflect local conditions or settings.
3. The decision based on a health **economic model** is obtained in an unambiguous, objective and transparent manner.
4. It allows the analyst to vary one or more parameter estimates, whose values might be uncertain, to see how the cost effectiveness ratio changes. This is referred to as **sensitivity analysis** (see Chapter 7) and will be discussed in more detail in the text that follows.

Suppose that we were uncertain about how effective treatment A really is. The typical scenario is that one clinical trial might report 60% of patients to be successfully treated, whereas another might report a higher value of 75%. A simple procedure, called univariate sensitivity analysis, can be applied by increasing the value of p from 0.6 to 0.75. When this is done, we notice that the incremental cost utility ratio increases to £91 250 per QALY, making first-line therapy with drug B much less attractive – the more effective drug A is, the more expensive drug B becomes per additional unit of benefit obtained.

And what about if we were uncertain about many (or all?) of the parameters listed in Table 9.1? One method is to vary each parameter in turn, as described above. Alternatively, more parameters can be varied at once by means of a bivariate or multivariate sensitivity analysis.

REPRESENTING UNCERTAINTY IN COST EFFECTIVENESS EVALUATIONS

More complex statistical procedures, including **Monte Carlo** simulations (which will be described in some detail), **bootstrapping** techniques and Fieller's theorem method (Glick et al 2001) are becoming more widely used to account for parameter uncertainty.

The process of performing a Monte Carlo simulation involves the repeated simulation of the model, each time drawing a different set of values from the sampling distribution of the model parameters, the results of which is a set of possible outcomes (outputs). This enables the generation of a distribution of expected costs and outcomes, which reflect the uncertainty of the parameter estimates. The deterministic model described thus far will now be modified to a stochastic model (one which considers parameter uncertainty) and analysed by Monte Carlo simulation.

To perform Monte Carlo simulations the sampling distribution of the model parameters (inputs) must be defined in advance, for example a normal distribution would be characterised by a mean, μ, and variance, σ^2. This can be done by inspection and analysis of patient level data. Other distributions, frequently used for Monte Carlo simulations, are listed below:

- Beta distribution: often used for binomial data, e.g. treatment is successful or unsuccessful (Fig. 9.3). It is characterised by two parameters, a and b, which can be thought of as counts of the event of interest versus its

Concept box 9.3 – Uncertainty analysis

There are a number of sources of uncertainty:
- parameter uncertainty: when the true numerical values of the parameters used as inputs are unknown
- model structure uncertainty: uncertainty about the correct method for combining parameters
- model process uncertainty: uncertainty in the entire process by which the analysis was completed by the analyst.

All forms must be considered when conducting or appraising an economic model. For parameter uncertainty, statistical methods such as bootstrapping and Monte Carlo simulation methods can be used to generate confidence intervals around the cost effectiveness estimate, or to generate cost effectiveness acceptability curves. Bootstrapping is a non-parametric method that takes into account the skewness of data and is thus primarily useful when distributions around a given parameter are skewed or when sample sizes are modest. Uncertainty analysis, based on Monte Carlo simulations, requires that the distributional forms of the parameters are specified. Both techniques involve several thousand replications, using a computer, to generate cost effectiveness estimates from which confidence intervals or cost effectiveness acceptability curves can be generated.

Concept box 9.4 – Monte Carlo simulation methods

This term was introduced by von Neumann and Ulam during their top-secret work on the atomic bomb at Los Alamos during World War II as a tongue-in-cheek reference to the gambling casinos in Monte Carlo.

Concept box 9.5 – Poisson probability

The Poisson probability is the probability that x number of events will occur over a given time period.

complement. For example, in a trial where 21 of 35 patients were treated successfully, a beta distribution with beta (21,14) (see Table 9.1) would be appropriate.
- Poisson distribution and gamma distributed mean: costs, which can be considered as a mixture of resource counts and unit costs, can be modelled by assuming a mixture of Poisson distribution with a gamma

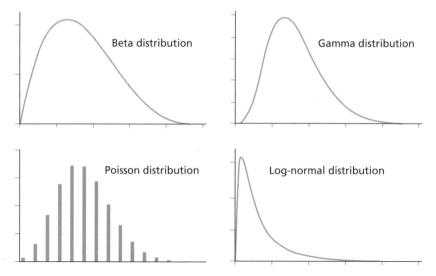

Fig 9.3 Probability distributions commonly used in pharmacoeconomic modelling. The plots represent the probability of an event occurring against the value of that particular event. In the case of costs being modelled by a log normal distribution, the distribution represents the probability that a particular cost, from zero to infinity, is incurred

distributed mean (a skewed, non-negative distribution) (Fig. 9.3). A popular alternative is to fit a log normal distribution to the cost data. This accounts for the fact that costs cannot be negative and are skewed, because a small number of patients often incur large costs. A log normal distribution accounts for this by being always positive and by having a slowly decreasing right tail.

- Log transformed relative risks can also be assumed to follow a log normal distribution.
- Utilities range in value from $-\infty$ (in theory) to +1. If negative utilities (states worse than death) are ignored then we can reasonably assume a beta distribution, otherwise we can fit a gamma or log normal distribution to the parameter x where $x = 1 -$ utility.

The third column in Table 9.1 lists the distributions assigned to each model parameter input. These allow a stochastic model to be constructed. The probabilities of treatment success and utility scores are assumed to follow beta distributions; costs associated with drug failure are represented by log normal distributions. The mean cost of successful treatment with drug A, for example, is $e^{5.3} = £200$.

Now that distributions have been assigned to each input parameter, the model is replicated a thousand or more times, drawing a sample at random from each distribution. In practice, this can be done with a computer using a conventional spreadsheet package or more specialised decision-analysis software. Each replication generates an **incremental cost** (cost associated with first-line therapy with drug B less the cost of stepped care) and an incremental outcome (QALYs associated with first-line therapy with drug B less the QALYs of stepped care). These can be plotted on the **cost effectiveness plane** (Fig. 9.4) to visualise the uncertainty in the cost effectiveness estimate.

There is a wide scatter in the distribution of the results, reflecting the uncertainty associated with the input parameter estimates. Most points appear in the north-east quadrant, suggesting the likelihood is that using drug B as first-line therapy is more effective but more expensive, overall, than the stepped-care approach. Some points, however, appear in the other quadrants. The incremental cost effectiveness ratio is not an appropriate measure of cost effectiveness in this instance for two reasons:

1. As the difference between the effectiveness of the two treatment pathways approaches zero (i.e. they are equally effective), the denominator approaches infinity.
2. Negative incremental cost effectiveness ratios, which occur for those points in the north-west and south-east quadrants of the cost effectiveness plane, make little intuitive sense and are not very helpful from a policy- or decision-making **perspective**.

Rather than thinking about ICERs to summarise the results of Fig. 9.4, the currently accepted method of analysis is to consider the probability of a treatment strategy being cost effective. Suppose that a decision maker's maximum **willingness to pay** (ceiling ratio) for a healthcare intervention is £30 000 per QALY. Now consider a line being drawn through the intercept with a slope equalling £30 000 per QALY. The proportion of points falling below that line represents the probability of the intervention being acceptable to the decision maker at the specified ceiling ratio. If this were repeated for a range of values for the ceiling ratio, with each corresponding probability of

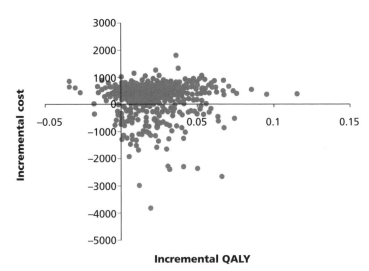

Fig 9.4 Cost effectiveness plane for the use of drug B as first-line therapy versus its use in a stepped-care approach in patients in whom drug A has failed

being cost effective plotted in turn, then a **cost effectiveness acceptability curve** is generated, as in Fig. 9.5.

Cost effectiveness acceptability curves facilitate the interpretation of analyses that incorporate parameter uncertainty. It enables the decision maker to ascertain the probability that a treatment strategy (in this example, the use of drug B as first-line therapy) is acceptable for any given value of ceiling ratio. Here, given a ceiling ratio of £30 000 per QALY gained, the probability that drug B is the most cost effective option is 60%. It is up to the decision maker now to decide whether this is too risky – the fact that there is a 40% chance that a stepped-care approach is more cost effective might be viewed as not being acceptable.

Bootstrapping. An alternative method for generating cost effectiveness acceptability curves is by using a resampling technique called bootstrapping. This technique is a non-parametric method and no assumptions are made about the underlying distribution of the cost and benefit data. The technique requires the mean of a sample, drawn at random with replacement, of paired cost and effect data to be calculated over and over again (a thousand times or more). These can be plotted on a cost effectiveness plane, as before, and used to construct a cost effectiveness acceptability curve. The main advantage of this method is that it does not require the underlying distributional forms of the data to be specified.

Fieller's theorem method. This is a parametric method that is based on the assumption that the differences in costs and the differences in benefits follow a bivariate normal distribution. Non-parametric bootstrapping and Fieller's theorem are now accepted as the most appropriate methods for estimating confidence intervals for incremental cost effectiveness ratios.

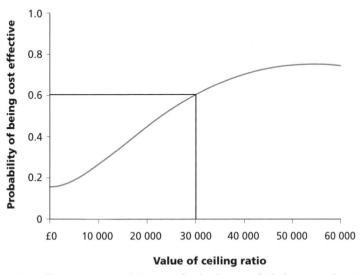

Fig 9.5 Cost effectiveness acceptability curve for the decision of whether to use drug B as first-line therapy or as part of a stepped-care approach

Linking intermediate clinical end-points to final outcomes

The other applications of modelling in pharmacoeconomics are related to instances where clinical trials have only measured intermediate end-points or short-term follow-up. Most clinical trials report drug action on a surrogate marker of efficacy. In the therapeutics of HIV, for example, drug effect on CD4 counts or viral load are often reported instead of survival and quality of life. Although these can be justified in terms of the requirements for drug registration and market approval, they are not ideal when decisions on healthcare resource allocations are required. A cost per percentage decrease in viral load, secondary to antiretroviral therapy, cannot be compared with a cost per life year gained, secondary to treatment with HMG CoA reductase inhibitors, unless a link is made between the intermediate end-point (in this case viral load) and survival. Mathematical models aimed at doing just this are frequently used. These are invariably based on epidemiological evidence and are used to link, for example, bone density and fractures, low-density lipoprotein cholesterol and survival, or glycosylated haemoglobin and the occurrence of diabetic complications.

We must be confident, however, that the link is clearly established and that a drug-induced change in the intermediate end-point can also be expected to occur in the final outcome. An example where this was not the case was in the Cardiac Arrhythmias Suppression Trial (CAST), where suppression of ventricular premature beats (VPBs) by use of the antiarrhythmic agent flecainide was hypothesised to reduce mortality in postmyocardial infarction patients (suppression of arrhythmias was thought to be a valid surrogate end-point for the avoidance of sudden cardiac death). It transpired that, rather than reducing mortality, the incidence of sudden cardiac death increased. Thus, although VPBs were adequately suppressed by flecainide, this effect did not translate to improvements in survival; suppression of VPBs was dismissed as a reliable surrogate marker of efficacy.

The longitudinal survey of residents of Framingham, Massachusetts, which was initiated in 1948 to study the factors associated with the development of cardiovascular disease by employing long-term surveillance of an adult population, provided a wealth of information on the links between various types of intermediary end-points and long-term outcomes. The survey was used to formulate prediction equations for several cardiovascular disease end-points, based on measurements of several known risk factors. Equations were developed to predict risk for myocardial infarction, coronary heart disease (CHD), death from CHD, stroke, cardiovascular disease and death from cardiovascular disease. The parametric models derived can provide predictions for different lengths of time and are archetypal examples of mathematical formulations of linking intermediate end-points and clinical outcomes, and of predicting future outcomes from short-term data. Morris (1997) compared the cost effectiveness estimates for cholesterol-modifying drugs from models, based on CHD risk equations taken from the Framingham Heart Study, with estimates based on trial evidence (the West of Scotland Coronary Prevention Study). The incremental cost per life year gained was comparable with both forms of analyses.

GENERALISING FROM ONE SETTING TO ANOTHER

Models are also used to generalise results from one setting to another, and from one country to another. Patients participating in clinical trials, for example, are far more compliant than patients in the 'real world'. For lipid-lowering therapy, which is intended to be life long, 5-year persistence rates of 13% have been reported. The results of a clinical trial are therefore unlikely to be generalisable to the general population. Models can be used to predict what might be the impact of poor compliance on therapeutic outcome by, for example, assuming that the patients who discontinue prematurely experience the same health benefits as patients who had been randomised to the placebo arm of a clinical trial (Hughes 2002).

Medical practices vary from place to place. The flexibility offered by decision analytic models allows for different treatment strategies to be incorporated into the analysis. Thus, for the example illustrated earlier, a different practice or HMO might also have drug C on their formulary, which might also be used when drug A fails. Models are also useful when extrapolating across different countries. As healthcare systems differ between countries, care must be exercised when applying the results of an economic evaluation to a different country. By considering these differences, and the differences likely to be encountered in the costs of healthcare interventions, models allow the user to explore such issues. It should always be remembered that drugs that are cost-effective in one country might not necessarily be cost-effective in another.

MODELLING DISEASE PROCESSES: MARKOV MODELS

One particularly suited application of modelling in the field of clinical decision analysis is to model the progression of chronic diseases (Briggs & Sculpher 1998). Decision analytic models, described earlier, are generally very static in that events occur at a single point in time. **Markov models** allow the analyst to model changes in the progression of disease over time. This requires the disease in question to be divided into distinct states, which are chosen to represent clinically and economically important events in the disease process. They should also be mutually exclusive because a patient cannot be in more than one health state simultaneously.

A simple example would be the following states: free from disease, mildly symptomatic, moderately severe, severe and death (Fig. 9.6). Movement of patients into and out of such states, over a discrete period of time (a Markov cycle), is determined by a set of transition probabilities. It is likely that untreated patients might progress from a milder form of the disease to a more severe form, over time. Equally possible are transitions from more severe to less severe states, for example when the disease is in remission. Drug therapies are clearly aimed at reducing the probability of disease progression and/or increasing the probability of remission. Certain states, such as death, are referred to as 'absorbing states' because they are impossible to leave.

Concept box 9.6 – Markov models

Markov models are particularly suited to modelling repeated events (e.g. headache) or the progression of chronic disease (e.g. multiple sclerosis). In a Markov model, the disease in question is divided into a finite set of health states, and individuals can move between health states over a discrete period of time according to a set of transition probabilities. By attaching estimates of resource use and outcomes (e.g. utilities) to each health state, and running the model over a long period of time (e.g. a lifetime), it is possible to generate long-term costs and outcomes for hypothetical cohorts of patients receiving treatments for a particular disease.

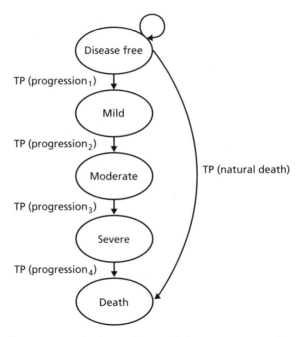

Fig 9.6 An illustrative example of a Markov model showing progression through the disease states until eventual death. Transition probabilities (TP) govern the movement of hypothetical cohorts of patients from one health state to the next

Probabilities for the natural progression of the disease are normally derived from longitudinal epidemiological surveys of diseased patients. Individual patient-level data from clinical trials are used to estimate the effect of the drug at each level of disease severity (health state).

A key feature of Markov models is the attaching of estimates of resource use and health outcomes to each state in the model. The model is then run over a large number of cycles and the total cost and outcome are obtained by summing across those cycles. This enables estimates of long-term costs and outcomes associated with a disease and a particular healthcare intervention to be determined.

If we consider multiple sclerosis as an example, health states can be divided according to scores on a specific measurement of impairment, such as the Expanded Disability Status Scale (EDSS). For convenience, categories of EDSS scores can be defined: 0 (normal functioning), 1–3, 4–6, 7–9 and 10 (death). Movement among health states are defined by transition probabilities, for example, left untreated, the probability of patients deteriorating from the second health state (EDSS score 1–3) to the third (EDSS score 4–6) over 1 year might be 0.3. This might be reduced to 0.25 with treatment. Health state 2 might be associated with a utility value of 0.75 and cost of £3000, compared with 0.55 and £4000, respectively, for state 3. As the model is run over a large number of cycles (e.g. 20 cycles, each of 1 year in duration) patients move among health states and accrue utilities and costs until, eventually, they all die. The total number of utilities, costs and years of survival are then used for cost-per-QALY calculations. Clearly both costs and benefits require **discounting** if the model exceeds 1 year in duration (see Chapter 7 on discounting).

Markov models are particularly useful when they are conducted using Monte Carlo simulation. Here, each subject in a hypothetical cohort is essentially treated as an individual and can be assigned very specific characteristics, such as age or presence of risk factor. The difference between the two methods is that although individual patients are subject to the same transition probabilities as the cohort of patients, they might or might not transit among states in any given cycle. Following the patient through the model allows an overall profile of costs and outcomes to be generated for that patient. Repeating the simulation a thousand or more times yields the distinct advantage of generating an estimate of the likely variance associated with the parameters estimated by the model. This uncertainty represents the inherent uncertainty of the probabilistic structure of the model.

GOOD MODELLING PRACTICE

If economic models are to be relied upon for clinical decision making, Buxton et al (1997) recommend five points for consideration, which are summarised in Box 9.1.

There will be a continued demand for analysts to produce economic models for use as tools to support clinical decision making. As the techniques upon which they rely are continuously being developed and improved, a parallel increased awareness and understanding of the techniques by end-users is essential. Some are sceptical of the assumptions made in economic models, and demand that attempts are made to validate results by conducting, where possible, appropriate trials. Others consider models as unavoidable facts of life (Buxton et al 1997) and argue that the real validation is in comparing and contrasting decisions informed, or otherwise, by the results of economic modelling. A randomised trial of informed versus uninformed decisions has yet to be conducted.

Box 9.1   Main considerations for good economic modelling practice

- The model should be kept as simple as possible to aid understanding by decision makers
- The presentation of the results from a model should be as transparent as possible, and the model itself should be made available for scrutiny
- A model (or for that matter any form of economic evaluation) is only as good as the data used for its construction. Data cannot simply be invented. Analysts often rely on expert opinion if 'hard data' are unavailable. In such circumstances, the analyst is responsible for making this clear to decision makers
- Through the process of modelling, the analyst should explore uncertainty rather than compensate for it. The robustness of the results should be tested by making thorough use of sensitivity analysis. Care should also be taken to avoid misrepresenting the decision at hand, for example, relevant alternative therapies cannot be ignored
- Models should be validated by comparing with other models, or by prospectively conducting an appropriate trial. The findings of economic evaluations require updating as and when new information is made available.

REFERENCES

Briggs A, Sculpher M 1998 An introduction to Markov modelling for economic evaluation. Pharmacoeconomics 13:397–409

Buxton M J, Drummond M F, Van Hout B A et al 1997 Modelling in economic evaluation: an unavoidable fact of life. Health Economics 6:217–227

Glick H A, Briggs A H, Polsky D 2001 Quantifying stochastic uncertainty and presenting results of cost effectiveness analyses. Expert Reviews in Pharmacoeconomics Outcomes Research 1:25–36

Hughes D A 2002 Economic impact of poor compliance with pharmaceuticals. Expert Reviews in Pharmacoeconomics Outcomes Research 2:327–335

Morris S 1997 A comparison of economic modelling and clinical trials in the economic evaluation of cholesterol-modifying pharmacotherapy. Health Economics 6:589–601

Nuijten M J C 1998 The selection of data sources for use in modelling studies. Pharmacoeconomics 13:305–316

Quality assurance in pharmacoeconomic analyses

10

EVALUATING PHARMACOECONOMIC STUDIES – 'SORTING THE WHEAT FROM THE CHAFF'

Healthcare professionals are increasingly exposed to pharmacoeconomic analyses to influence their decision making on, for instance, drug choice for formularies. Ensuring that only the most beneficial drugs gain access to the formulary is essential to ensure appropriate and rational prescribing (National Prescribing Centre 1998). These analyses require access to high-quality evidence concerning both the clinical and cost effectiveness of any new drug. In addition, subgroup analyses should be undertaken where necessary to ensure that new drugs can be effectively targeted on patients who might benefit to the greatest degree.

A large number of critical appraisal skill programmes are incorporated into clinical epidemiology courses to assist the reader to appraise the clinical literature. This chapter aims to provide non-specialists with similar tools to appraise the quality of published pharmacoeconomic studies and assess the extent to which they are robust and reliable enough to alter their clinical practice. In addition, those who perform such studies need guidance about what factors should be addressed if they are to meet the best critical appraisal of their work. Appendix 1 is the checklist provided to authors submitting a **health economics** paper to the **British Medical Journal**.

Concept box 10.1 – Tools of critical appraisal

Checklists
- Outline the attributes and standards exhibited by good quality studies

Guidelines
- Complimentary approach to use of checklists
- Attempt to ensure that studies at least conform to a minimum acceptable standard.

155

EVALUATING PUBLISHED PHARMACOECONOMIC ANALYSES – USING CHECKLISTS

One method of supporting the critical interpretation of pharmacoeconomic analyses is through the use of a checklist that outlines the attributes and standards that should be expected from good studies and many such checklists have been published (see, for example, Appendix 2). It is important to emphasise that not all studies will, or should, meet all of the criteria in a checklist, but its use will assist in directing the critical facilities of the non-specialist to the specific elements in a pharmacoeconomic analysis that would be most likely to determine its quality. In addition, such checklists aim to improve the overall quality of pharmacoeconomic analyses produced. The proper aim of such analyses is not just to alter the pattern of prescribing in favour of the drug being evaluated but to help prescribers to improve the clinical and economic **effectiveness** of their prescribing behaviour for the benefit of patients.

A number of methods can be used to introduce a degree of bias into pharmacoeconomic analyses and undermine the reliability of the results. Appendix 3 ('A crook's guide to pharmacoeconomic analysis') takes a light-hearted look at some of these biases. Underlying this 'crook's' guide, however, is a serious issue: as health professionals become more aware of quality markers in pharmacoeconomic analyses, they will increasingly refuse to be influenced by poor-quality or biased studies. Such studies will no longer be undertaken because they will have no persuasive value and will increasingly reflect badly on the sponsoring companies. They will be replaced by analyses that are persuasive because they provide objective high-quality scientific pharmacoeconomic evidence, which can be incorporated into local decision-making processes. The following checklist (Haycox & Walley 1997) is therefore one way to increase the expectations of health professionals and hopefully improve the quality of such analyses in the future. Two case studies addressing the practical application of the checklist to papers analyzing the cost effectiveness of thrombolysis and cholesterol lowering drugs are provided in Appendices 4 and 5.

Question 1. Is the question appropriate?

Issues to be addressed include:

- Is a clear hypothesis provided?
- Can this hypothesis be tested?
- Is it relevant and appropriate to the real world?

For example, a question such as, 'Is drug A cost effective?' is incomplete because it does not recognise that the cost effectiveness of any intervention depends upon what it is being compared with. A more appropriate question would be, 'Is drug A more cost effective than drug B?' It is then necessary to identify how relevant this question actually is. For example, if the comparison is with a subtherapeutic dosage of an obsolete therapy, the question might be inappropriate (see question 4).

> **Concept box 10.2 – Evaluating the health economics literature**
>
> 1. Is the question appropriate?
> 2. From what perspective is the study undertaken?
> 3. Is the methodology appropriate?
> 4. Is the comparator appropriate?
> 5. Is the evaluation based on good quality clinical evidence?
> 6. Are appropriate costs and benefits considered?
> 7. Is differential timing taken into account?
> 8. Is a marginal analysis undertaken?
> 9. Is a sensitivity analysis undertaken?
> 10. Is the analysis appropriate to the local environment?

Question 2. From what perspective is the study undertaken?

Issues to be addressed include:

- Was the **perspective** clearly specified?
- Was it from a societal perspective?
- Was it from a health service perspective?

Ideally, studies should evaluate the impact of changes in resource use from an overall societal perspective, rather than a more limited perspective (e.g. that of the health service alone). However, although a societal perspective could provide the most comprehensive analysis of costs and benefits, a narrower range of viewpoints might be of value to decision makers in certain circumstances (e.g. isolating the impact of any change upon the pharmaceutical budget). In practice, the perspective adopted by any study often depends on the question being addressed and the budgetary responsibility of the decision maker. In the UK, for instance, NICE requires that pharmacoeconomic analyses look beyond NHS costs and consider the implications on other publicly funded resources such as social services.

The crucial factor is that the perspective underlying the analysis, and a justification of its selection, must be specified clearly. In cases where studies use a limited perspective (health service or even the resource implications for the individual hospital) the justification for, and the implications of, restricting the perspective must be addressed together with consideration of the costs and benefits that are likely to fall outside the chosen perspective.

Question 3. Is the methodology appropriate?

Issues to be addressed include:

- Was the methodology appropriate given the nature and context of the analysis being carried out?

- Was the implicit treatment of outcome variations that underlie the choice of methodology appropriate to the clinical comparison being made?

The method chosen depends on the nature of the comparison being undertaken, and on the way in which benefits are measured (see Chapter 7). In such circumstances, the chosen method automatically defines a relationship between the clinical outcomes between the drugs being compared. The nature of this relationship is defined below:

- **Cost minimisation analysis (CMA)**: the benefits of the interventions are identical, e.g. comparing the costs of a generic drug and branded drug, providing they are bioequivalent.
- **Cost effectiveness analysis (CEA)**: the benefits are common, unidimensional and measured in the same natural units, e.g. comparing the number of deaths prevented by coronary artery bypass with the number prevented by use of a statin.
- **Cost utility analysis (CUA)**: benefits are multidimensional, including measurement of both quantity and quality of life, e.g. comparing the number of **quality-adjusted-life years** (QALYs) gained by use of a statin with those gained by a hip replacement.
- **Cost benefit analysis (CBA)**: benefits are valued in monetary units, e.g. comparing the amount of money one is willing to pay to prevent a death by instituting either a breast-screening programme or a cervical-screening programme.

This is one of the areas in which it is most important that health professionals apply their therapeutic judgement and clinical knowledge. For example, if they feel that significant variations do occur in the benefits provided by two drugs compared in a cost minimisation analysis, then they fundamentally reject the basic assumption on which the choice of methodology was made and hence need not consider the analysis any further. In this manner, pharmacoeconomic analyses enhance rather than replace the need for clinical judgement.

Question 4. Is the comparator appropriate?

- If the evaluation addresses a new drug, the comparator should be the 'gold standard' intervention used in the country in which the analysis is being undertaken.
- Is the comparator being used at an optimal therapeutic dose?
- If a 'gold standard' comparator is not used, does the reader feel that the reasons underlying the choice of an alternative comparator are sufficiently justified and clinically reasonable?

The choice of comparator will fundamentally affect the results obtained and hence the interpretation of the comparative cost effectiveness of any drug. If the comparator is chosen from a generation of drugs no longer widely used, or the comparator is used at a subtherapeutic dose, then it will inevitably improve the apparent 'cost effectiveness' of the new drug being evaluated. Therefore, before analysing the results of a pharmacoeconomic study in detail, readers must assume that the comparison is appropriate to their clinical practice and that the reasons underlying the choice of comparator are justified and considered to be reasonable.

Medical practice varies widely between countries. A comparator felt to be reasonable for a study based in one country might not be appropriate for another. The comparator chosen must be a reasonable alternative in the country where the analysis is being performed.

Question 5. Is the evaluation based on good quality clinical evidence?

Issues to be addressed by the reader include:

- Is there good quality evidence that the intervention is clinically effective?
- Does the health economic evaluation use these data as a basis for the analysis?
- Are the interventions compared within the same trial?
- If not, are the studies conducted in similar patient groups over a similar timeframe and with similar outcome measures that enable indirect comparisons to be meaningful?

A critical issue underlying any health economic evaluation is the degree to which the clinical evidence is available and accurate (Haycox & Walley 1997). The extent to which clinical trial data can be used to inform health economic analyses is often a matter of judgement.

Ideally, the costs and benefits arising from two drugs should be compared within the same trial. However, it is often necessary to use indirect evidence by combining results from separate trials. In such circumstances, the selective identification of trials favourable to one drug might be used to bias the clinical evidence underlying health economic studies (Box 10.1). It is essential to ensure that pharmacoeconomic analyses are based upon a balanced view of the available clinical evidence.

Question 6. Are appropriate costs and benefits considered?

Issues to be addressed include:

- Have **opportunity costs** been considered?

Box 10.1   Case example – the cost effectiveness of an SSRI

A published cost effectiveness analysis of a selective serotonin reuptake inhibitor (SSRI) antidepressant was based on a single trial, which rather atypically showed a large benefit for that agent. However, when the results of this study were incorporated with several other studies in a meta-analysis, the benefits perceived from the studies as a whole were much smaller. This showed that the cost effectiveness of the SSRI had been overestimated as a consequence of basing the effectiveness side of the analysis on the results of a single atypical study (Freemantle & Maynard 1994).

- Is the evaluation flexible enough to take account of local variations in practice?
- Are all patients in the clinical trial involved in the economic analysis?

Many different types of cost should be considered in a good-quality health economic evaluation (see Chapter 7). The true cost incurred in treating one patient is the unavailability of resources to treat another (opportunity cost). Within a fixed budget, any increased cost associated with a treatment can only be met by an overall reduction in the number of patients treated. This missed opportunity to benefit patients is the basis of the concept of the opportunity cost. Many evaluations fail to consider the benefits that would have arisen by using the resources allocated to the intervention under consideration in an alternative manner (e.g. to prevent the onset of the disease through health promotion strategies).

To enable the reader to judge the validity of the approach taken, the perspective and methods used to measure both costs and benefits must be transparent. Pharmacoeconomic evaluations must also be flexible enough to take account of local variations in clinical practice or resources. The effect of such variations can be encompassed either directly, by incorporating the impact of local practice and prices into the analysis, or by doing a **sensitivity analysis** to assess the extent to which such variations change the overall results (see later).

The costs and benefits of drug therapy on all patients should be analysed, irrespective of whether they are responders, non-responders or patients experiencing adverse drug reactions (Box 10.2).

Question 7. Is differential timing taken into account?

Issues to be addressed include:

- Have future costs and benefits been incorporated into the analysis?
- Have such costs and benefits been appropriately discounted?
- Have appropriate discount rates been used and, where appropriate, different analyses been undertaken, one using **discounting** and one not using discounting?

Therapeutic alternatives might have different time distributions of their costs and benefits. For example, the majority of costs related to surgery for cardiovascular disease are incurred immediately, while costs are ongoing for similar benefits with a drug therapy. In such cases, it is necessary to adjust the

---

Box 10.2 Case example – the cost effectiveness of a new asthma therapy

A relatively inexpensive new drug for asthma might produce a greater long-term improvement in pulmonary function than existing therapy. However, only a limited number of patients respond and many experience serious adverse effects, requiring hospitalisation. An economic evaluation of this drug that neglected to consider the costs associated with no response and with hospitalisation due to adverse effects, would possibly draw a false conclusion, i.e. that the drug is a cost effective option compared with existing therapy.

impact of future costs and benefits to their net present value (NPV). The role of discounting is discussed further in Chapter 7.

Although most health economists accept the need to discount future health costs, the discounting of future health benefits is more controversial. Health economic studies should provide two measures of future health benefit, one discounted and one not. Evaluations in which the conclusions reached do not vary according to whether benefits are discounted will be more reliable than those that do.

Question 8. Is a marginal analysis undertaken?

Issues to be addressed include:

- Did the analysis relate to the provision of a new service (in which case **average costs** are appropriate) or a change in the scale of provision of a service (in which case **marginal costs** are appropriate)?
- Was the nature of the underlying cost function analysed?

Most therapeutic areas have an existing level of costs and benefits associated with them. When a new treatment is introduced, or services are contracted or expanded, there is a change in the overall costs and benefits. As the relationship between costs and benefits is rarely linear, these marginal costs and benefits should be made explicit within the health economic analysis.

Marginal costs will vary from average costs in cases where certain costs are relatively fixed in the short-term and will not vary in response to a small increase or reduction in treatment. A drug that saves 10 minutes of nurse time as a consequence of simplified administration will exert little influence upon nurse staffing in the short-term. However, where the drug is widely used, its impact upon nursing workload could facilitate a reallocation of nursing tasks over a longer time period. The results of marginal analyses are frequently presented in the form of an incremental cost effectiveness ratio (ICER), which compares marginal cost changes with marginal changes in effectiveness. The way in which the ICER is calculated is discussed in Chapter 7.

The estimate of marginal costs depends not only on the nature of changes in resource use but also on the extent of such changes and the time period being analysed. When targeting drug therapy, it is important to recognise that the marginal costs and benefits generated by any therapeutic intervention can vary significantly between the different subgroups.

Question 9. Is a sensitivity analysis undertaken?

Issues to be addressed include:

- Was a range of likely costs and benefits given?
- Were the assumptions made within the evaluation made explicit and transparent?
- Were the limitations and weaknesses of the analysis made clear by the authors?

The key parameters underlying pharmacoeconomic analyses must be subject to a sensitivity analysis. Accurate point estimates of costs and benefits are seldom possible and an analysis that is robust within a realistic range of costs and benefits is likely to be more reliable. For example, if drug A is identified as being cost effective compared to drug B at current prices, what happens if the comparative price of the drugs changes? Can we identify the break-even price to which drug B will have to be reduced for it to become as cost effective as drug A?

The use of sensitivity analysis also enables the reader to identify the critical assumptions upon which the conclusions are based and, therefore, which assumptions require confirmation. For instance, where a study assumes that a drug used to treat dyspepsia requires only 25% of patients to undergo gastroscopy, do the overall conclusions still stand if this rises to 50%? If the results of such sensitivity analyses are not reported, it is impossible to assess the robustness and hence the reliability of the results.

Question 10. Is the analysis appropriate to the local environment?

Issues to be addressed include:

- Are the costs used in the analysis similar to the costs of services locally?
- Are the clinical data underpinning the economic evaluation applicable to local clinical practice?
- Are the resources used in the analysis available locally?

Pharmacoeconomic analysis are only of value if they are presented in a manner that helps to inform clinical decision making. For example, if pharmaco-economic analysis compares the cost effectiveness of drug therapy and surgery, to what extent can the results be transferred and generalised to an environment in which the local costs associated with surgery are lower than those assumed in the study? To apply such analyses to local circumstances, it is necessary to apply local unit costs and local clinical practice within the context of the pharmacoeconomic analysis. Studies that report quantities of resources separately from the total cost lend themselves more easily to clinical decision making at a local level.

EVALUATING ECONOMIC MODELS – KEY PRINCIPLES

Increasingly, pharmacoeconomic analyses involve economic modelling (see Chapter 9). When evaluating the quality of pharmacoeconomic models, similar critical appraisal principles apply. It is equally important to be able to distinguish a high-quality science-based model from one that has largely been produced as a marketing tool (Sheldon 1996). Given the wide variety of factors, which vary from place to place, pharmacoeconomic analyses should ideally be interactive, allowing the user to tailor them to local needs. The ability to introduce local costs and clinical practices into an **economic model** is increasingly an essential aspect of pharmacoeconomic modelling as it enhances the local value and applicability of such studies.

Aspects of good modelling practice are discussed in Chapter 9 and include (Buxton et al 1997):

- keeping the model simple
- making the assumptions transparent
- presenting the results in a transparent manner
- being explicit about the quality of the data
- conducting adequate sensitivity analysis to eliminate major areas of uncertainty
- validating the work by comparing it with that of others in a similar area, to ensure consistency and reliability.

The quality of the clinical evidence underlying the economic model is crucial. Unfortunately, for many models the evidence base will be incomplete, inconclusive or contradictory. This inevitably requires assumptions to be made. Such assumptions must be transparent, objective and, where necessary, based on independent and high-quality expert opinion. The process by which expert opinion is incorporated into the analysis needs to be robust, credible and stated explicitly.

Transparency in model construction enables the quality and appropriateness of assumptions to be assessed and, where necessary, altered to reflect clinical reality or local circumstances. Openness requires models to be freely available to healthcare professionals and academics for validation and replication.

Both transparency and openness have implications for the documentation that must be produced in support of them. Both the model and user guide should be provided to enable a range of scenario analyses to be undertaken. Only by enabling local decision makers to gain familiarity with the structure and assumptions underlying the model, and allowing them to alter the model to better reflect local circumstances, will they gain ownership of the model in a manner that allows them to incorporate it into local decision-making processes.

PRACTICAL PROBLEMS WITH THE APPLICATION OF ECONOMIC EVALUATION TO HEALTHCARE SERVICES

Two issues not often debated in pharmacoeconomic evaluations are the questions of **affordability** and the issue of opportunity costs. Issues of affordability arise particularly when a particular therapy is highly cost effective but simply cannot be afforded from a fixed and highly constrained healthcare budget. In such circumstances, a cost-effective new drug might not be taken up simply because the resources required to fund it are simply not available. Similarly, pharmacoeconomic analyses are inevitably partial because they compare two options within the context of an overall system of healthcare. Proving that a drug provides sufficient additional benefits to justify its additional cost does not imply that it represents the best use of any additional resources available to local prescribers. If we accept that health services will never be able to fund all desirable new and innovative drugs, then we must also accept that they should attempt to focus not only on cost-effective new drugs but also on the most cost-effective new drugs. Thus, proving that a drug is cost effective (by some generally accepted definition) is a necessary but not sufficient element underlying its use; it should be prescribed only if it is the most cost-effective alternative use of the available healthcare funds. Again, the crucial economic concept of opportunity cost emphasises that a good new drug should not be allowed to pre-empt funds from the best new drug.

Pharmacoeconomic evaluations do not have a 'gold standard' methodology. As a result, they can be open to bias and distortion, particularly with respect to the choice of comparator, the nature of the assumptions made or the selective use of medical evidence. In overcoming poor-quality analyses, health economists must educate and collaborate closely with other health professionals (Kernick 1998) to ensure that decision makers are aware of the potential for, and sources of, bias (Friedberg et al 1999). Irrespective of their source, pharmacoeconomic evaluations must be appraised critically to ensure that they are of good quality, appropriate and relevant.

The journal in which the paper is published will provide an indication of its quality. A paper published in a journal that is known to have a rigorous process of peer review is likely to be of higher quality than one published in a journal that uses peer review less rigorously or not at all. Equally, the credibility of the authors of the analysis is just as important, especially with regard to their status and the independence of their funding. In this respect, however, it is important to recognise that many high-quality pharmacoeconomic analyses have been produced either directly by the pharmaceutical industry or using funding provided by the pharmaceutical industry. Conversely, an analysis produced by an independent academic or government unit should be appraised with equal rigour to assess its quality and appropriateness to the local decision-making environment. The current adherence in published papers to guidelines for economic analysis leaves room for progress (Briggs & Gray 1999), irrespective of their source.

CONCLUSION

Pharmacoeconomics is still in its infancy and is developing slowly as a speciality in its own right. The quality of its science can only be refined by application, and as the science improves so too will the value of health economic analyses to clinicians (Robinson 1993). Many economic evaluations are funded by pharmaceutical companies and are sometimes perceived to lack independent credibility. In many cases, such an assumption is unfair. Generally, if the science is good then, as in clinical studies, the funding for the research is of secondary importance. The crucial issue is for health professionals and the editors of journals publishing health economic papers, to be able to identify well-conducted studies.

More high-quality economic analyses will be carried out by commercially motivated suppliers of such data (i.e. the pharmaceutical industry) when customers (i.e. healthcare professionals) are confident in their ability to evaluate the quality of the underlying economic analyses. Poor quality and biased analyses will be of little value once healthcare professionals become more aware of the distinguishing characteristics of high-quality studies. Once this occurs, prescribers will come to demand higher-quality analyses to help inform (rather than distort) their decision making.

REFERENCES

Briggs A H, Gray A M 1999 Handling uncertainty in economic evaluations of healthcare interventions. British Medical Journal 319(7210):635–638

Buxton M J Drummond M F, Van Hout B A et al 1997 Modelling in economic evaluation: an unavoidable fact of life. Health Economics 6(3): 217–227

Freemantle N, Maynard A 1994 Something rotten in the state of clinical and economic evaluations? Health Economics 3(2): 63–77

Friedberg M, Saffran B, Stinson T J et al 1999 Evaluation of conflict of interest in economic analyses of new drugs used in oncology. Journal of the American Medical Association 282(15):1453–1457

Haycox A, Walley T 1997 Pharmacoeconomics: evaluating the evaluators. British Journal of Clinical Pharmacology 43(5): 451–456

Haycox A, Drummond M, Walley T 1997 Pharmacoeconomics: integrating economic evaluation into clinical trials. British Journal of Clinical Pharmacology 43(6): 559–562

Kernick D P 1998 Has health economics lost its way? British Medical Journal 317(7152): 197–199

National Prescribing Centre 1998 GP prescribing support. NHS Executive, London

Robinson R 1993 The policy context. British Medical Journal 307(6910): 994–996

Sheldon T A 1996 Problems of using modelling in the economic evaluation of health care. Health Economics 5(1):1–11

The future challenges

11

The future challenges facing **pharmacoeconomics** will spring from advances in two areas: first, the future nature and direction of national and European pharmaceutical policies and second, technical and other developments in the methods of pharmacoeconomic evaluation. The anticipated impact of both factors is considered in this concluding chapter.

CHALLENGES DERIVED FROM FUTURE PHARMACEUTICAL POLICY

Publicly funded health services across the world will inevitably become subject to mounting tension as they are caught between strict resource constraints and increased demands from demography, enhanced patient expectations and the expanding cost and availability of new drugs and other healthcare technologies. As the cost of health systems increases, it remains uncertain how willing societies will prove to be in maintaining an equitable and redistributive health service. Additional funding will be required, either in the form of increased taxation or extra social insurance payments. Future claims for additional funding for the health service might become overshadowed by the demands of an ageing population on other publicly funded services. However, the UK has for the moment decided to prioritise the needs of the health service by raising the level of funding devoted to the NHS. This might not be adequate in the long term and prioritisation of healthcare services seems to be inevitable.

It is vital that every country in the European Union debates and, wherever possible agrees upon, the finance, delivery and organisation of its domestic health services. At one extreme, it might be accepted that the health service should provide no more than a safety net for those who cannot pay for private health care; such changes would fundamentally alter the nature of healthcare in the UK and the services that patients have a 'right' to expect. Currently, however, it would appear that most Europeans would not relish the prospect of a fragmented US-style scheme of healthcare with the associated limitations in access. European societies appear to recognise and accept that the value of a healthcare system lies not only in its ability to provide care but also in the basis on which healthcare is actually provided. For example, the Royal

Commission on the NHS (1979) emphasised the many benefits derived by the people of the UK from being supported by a National Health Service that is free at the point of delivery. This psychological benefit manifests itself in a degree of loyalty and level of support for a healthcare system that is tampered with at politicians' peril.

The European Union is currently in the process of unifying disparate national licensing policies. With a single European market, there is pressure to reduce the wide disparity in prices across the EU. The parallel import trade already takes advantage of this and has largely been protected under EU law. Many countries are looking to NICE-type arrangements, wondering if they are all reinventing the wheel and debating whether there is a role for a Euro Institute for Clinical Excellence that could undertake clinical and cost effectiveness evaluations. Pan-European evaluations would have to be undertaken with caution. Whereas certain elements of the work that NICE does – the clinical assessment for instance –would be applicable across all member states, the economic evaluation and the health service impact analysis would be too closely bound up with the structure of each individual health service to be immediately transferable without modification.

Cost containment is a key focus of any pharmaceutical policy. Issues relating to cost containment are most immediately visible in relation to pharmaceutical expenditure because it represents the second largest cost to health services after salaries. However, although salary costs are normally seen as being sacrosanct (to prevent a reduction in the numbers of doctors and nurses), the same solidarity is not evident in support of drug budgets. The perception that excessive profits are being made by pharmaceutical companies ensures that they are viewed as a natural and easy target for cost containment measures. As drug therapy becomes more effective, and inevitably more expensive, it is perhaps both natural and desirable that it takes an increased share of the healthcare budget. As drugs evolve and are used to facilitate early discharge or substitute ambulatory for inpatient care, the need for hospital facilities (and their associated resources) might fall. However, the extent to which healthcare decision makers will grasp the nettle of shifting the focus of healthcare expenditure from staff to drugs remains to be seen.

In the past, prescribers have been, to a certain extent, protected from the immediate effects of central pressure to contain costs. However, the future impact of these pressures will become more direct as doctors are forced increasingly to confront budgetary limitations and the focus of power shifts from the individual doctor towards local prescribing committees or advisers. This will require healthcare planners to develop programme budgets that enable them to accrue resources and to reconfigure services so that the new therapies can be used to best advantage and that any savings available from the new therapy can be realised. Decision makers therefore need early warning and early evaluation, even if this is based on limited data with the evaluation being repeated at a later stage as better information becomes available. Unless such planning and evaluation occurs, pharmaceutical budgets will become overwhelmed by the new demands placed upon them, leading health services to resort to ad hoc 'coping strategies' (such as refusing to fund any new drugs), which would be both inefficient and inequitable.

The pharmaceutical industry also faces unprecedented challenges in the future. Successful companies will need to provide clinical and economic information to decision makers at an earlier stage in drug development and so will need to look carefully at how economic evaluation can dovetail into clinical trials and where pharmacoeconomic modelling can extrapolate costs and benefits accurately into longer-term and real-world contexts.

Already, pharmacoeconomic evaluations are being undertaken at an earlier stage (Phase II) in the drug development process. These can be of enormous value to determine the potential benefit of moving into the expensive Phase III stage and, where indicated, optimising future clinical and economic trial design. Given the importance of obtaining early evidence of cost effectiveness (ideally to be available at the time of product launch), such analyses should in the future become an integral part of each pharmaceutical company's drug development programme. One of the most important new approaches to obtaining such early information on cost effectiveness is by combining clinical trial simulation and health economic modelling. Such an approach uses the results of early pharmacoeconomic evaluations to lead to more informed 'go/no-go' decisions during the drug development process (Hughes & Walley 2001). This information is likely to become increasingly important in gaining market access and rapid market dissemination in a growing number of countries.

There is also a role for adopting the paradigms of 'learning' and 'confirming' to drug development. Phases I, II and IV are largely confined to learning about the actions of a drug (Phase IV about how it works in the real world), whereas Phase III is primarily concerned with confirming that which has been learnt at an earlier stage for regulatory purposes. Such a change in paradigm might lead to a change in emphasis from evaluations in phases I–III to more postmarketing safety and (cost) effectiveness studies in Phase IV, or to an even broader change in which orphan drugs are developed in public–private partnerships. This has already occurred to some extent with drugs such as the antimalarial mefloquine: the US government funded much of the early development but commercialisation was undertaken in collaboration with a pharmaceutical company. This might help reduce the considerable commercial risk associated with drug development, and also ensure that drug research will become refocused on areas of unmet need as governments will not be interested in funding research where there are already reasonable drug options. The use of pharmacoeconomic tools will improve companies' ability to assess the commercial risks that exist and will help governments to assess continued public funding for a particular line of drug development.

Finally, successful companies will have to deal with the anticipated reduction in the rate of new drugs in response to increased drug development costs. With fewer new drugs coming through most companies' pipelines, blockbusters will become increasingly rare in the future. New drugs are likely to be targeted more precisely on smaller numbers of patients with particular genetic profiles, leading to an inevitable rise in the unit costs of many drugs.

The greatest future challenge to pharmaceutical policy is to promote the development of effective and safe medicines while facilitating patients' access to them at an affordable cost. Part of this tension arises from the fact that many countries need to maintain a profitable and innovative domestic pharmaceutical industry. If health services are to take full advantage of the benefits of new medicines, some mechanism to balance these tensions in the future becomes essential. It is not possible for pharmacoeconomics alone to resolve these problems. However, one of the great strengths of pharmacoeconomics is that it can bring such issues into sharper focus for **stakeholders**, whereas previously these issues were often obfuscated. Pharmacoeconomics will increasingly play a leading role in assisting healthcare decision makers to make best use of their limited resources by informing their decision making. In particular, the UK National Institute for Clinical Excellence (see Chapter 3) is, and will continue to be, an important example of pharmacoeconomics in action and has an increasing ability to influence decision makers.

FUTURE TECHNICAL DEVELOPMENTS IN HEALTH ECONOMICS AND PHARMACOECONOMICS

It is important to remember that the discipline of pharmacoeconomics is still in its infancy and a wide range of fundamental, theoretical and practical issues remain to be resolved. The manner in which technical issues are addressed is likely to shape the future structure of pharmacoeconomics. In particular, a topic of major concern is the technical development and appropriate role of economic modelling within pharmacoeconomics.

Developments in economic modelling

A number of technical developments will underpin the role and scope of economic modelling in the future. Foremost among these is the need to develop a theoretical framework to guide the development of modelling techniques so as to delineate a more pragmatic approach to evidence synthesis and model construction. A number of such developments are outlined briefly below:

1. *Enhanced understanding of model selection and design.* At present, the majority of pharmacoeconomic models are limited by their use of methods most appropriately applied to relatively uncomplicated conditions of short duration. Increasingly, pharmacoeconomics will involve evaluation of new interventions in chronic and complex diseases that present particular problems not amenable to a single 'off-the-shelf' methodology. The choice of a particular model structure should be fundamentally related to a modeller's understanding of the medical condition and its natural history, the impact and consequences of the intervention, and also the nature of the evaluation being undertaken. Adoption of an inappropriate structure introduces into the analysis implicit assumptions about the problem that, at best, make the modeller's task more difficult and at worst might bias any results obtained. The continued development of checklists to aid the design and appraisal of

pharmacoeconomic models will be an enormous help in the efficient and effective development of new evaluation models.

2. *Enhanced understanding of pharmacoeconomic 'drivers'.* The notion of 'drivers' in pharmacoeconomic modelling is frequently misunderstood and misapplied. The essential quality of a successful model is its ability to resolve a complex situation into a relatively simple conceptual framework. In so doing, it aids understanding of the essence of decision making by integrating the various disparate elements through a comparatively small number of driving influences. In pharmacoeconomic modelling, this should mean that the most important features of the medical condition and the intervention(s) are linked directly to related incremental changes in the main outcome measures and the principle variable costs. Identification of such 'drivers' will generally allow results to be presented to decision makers in a simpler (but none the less valid) form. The driving elements should be identified at the design stage, thus improving the design of the model itself.

3. *Extrapolating beyond limited clinical evidence.* Increasingly, policy makers will be required to judge the appropriateness and desirability of adopting new drugs at a very early stage in the life cycle of each drug. Inevitably, at the time when these judgements are required, the evidence available for **efficacy** and **effectiveness** could be limited in both volume and duration. It is therefore important to further develop the alternative methods for estimating future effects from current evidence. These range from formal analytical procedures (such as time series analysis and forecasting), techniques borrowed from other disciplines (such as clinical trial simulations) to a more Bayesian approach of assigning prior probabilities of likely improvements in the technology itself, or in operator performance. Another key factor is the 'weight' afforded to different forms of clinical evidence, given that the hierarchy of evidence adopted for a pharmacoeconomic model might have a significant influence on the results obtained. Consideration must also be given to the relevance of various methods of synthesising data from different sources (e.g. clinical trials) by means other than traditional meta-analysis, and projecting them beyond their immediate validity.

4. *Future improvements in incorporating uncertainty into pharmacoeconomic modelling.* A great deal of research effort has been expended in improving statistical approaches to estimating the levels of uncertainty associated with the results obtained in pharmacoeconomic models. As data on cost, effectiveness and outcomes are commonly obtained from disparate sources then it is usual to construct an **economic model** to combine clinical trial information on effectiveness with other information on resource use and costs. Many of the parameters of such a model will not be known precisely but will be estimated from the various data sources. It is then necessary to quantify uncertainty on those parameters, and thereby to measure the uncertainty on outputs of interest such as net health benefits. There is considerable and growing interest in the use of Bayesian statistics for this kind of analysis because, arguably, it makes explicit the assumptions relating to uncertainty. Under a Bayesian interpretation, parameters of interest are ascribed a distribution reflecting uncertainty concerning the true value of the parameter.

Bayesian methods might usefully be classified into three main types, depending on the approach to prior information:

- Empirical Bayes describes the approach of estimating prior distributions on the basis of previously available statistical information.
- A second approach to Bayes would be to assume no information concerning the parameter of interest.
- The third approach could be described as subjective Bayes, where prior information is elicited from experts on the basis of their personal beliefs.

However, there are reasons to question whether such an approach provides useful information for the decision maker. First, in a model of any degree of complexity the additional information required (in terms of probability distributions) normally far exceeds the empirical evidence available, so that the results obtained are heavily dependent on a large number of additional assumptions. Second, **Monte Carlo** simulation is only feasible for a restricted number of model structures, and third, this approach can be very demanding in computational time and is not readily amenable to external verification, leaving decision makers with little option but to take findings 'on trust'. The current emphasis on Monte Carlo simulation is therefore open to challenge.

Given the inevitability of uncertainty in pharmacoeconomic models, it is essential that increasingly sophisticated methods for dealing with this factor be developed in the future. In particular, other approaches to assessing the reliability of models should be explored (e.g. different types of **sensitivity analysis**) to assess the extent to which they are better able to determine the robustness of pharmacoeconomic analyses.

5. Life cycle modelling of new technologies. New technologies tend to be initially expensive but become cheaper over time. Also, in many cases experience can improve performance of the technology itself, or the way it is employed. In the future it will become increasingly important to assess the extent to which it is legitimate to combine time-profile projections with current evidence in evaluating the impact and benefits of healthcare innovations.

6. Incorporating pragmatic factors in models –moving from efficacy to effectiveness. It is common for drugs with high efficacy reported in clinical trials to disappoint users when employed in ordinary clinical practice. Several factors contribute to this effect, including patient non-compliance, physician misprescribing and the social or environmental context. Policy makers now and in the future need to base their decisions on the clinical and economic benefits that arise in practice rather than on the narrow and unrealistic confines of a clinical trial.

7. Relationship between isolated technology evaluation and 'in situ' policy impact modelling. Assessing the technical efficiency of a new treatment does not necessarily provide local planners with appropriate information on which to judge priorities for service development. The relative local state of the various elements contributing to healthcare for the target patient group constitutes a unique decision-making context and means that the marginal cost effectiveness of any decision will vary from place to place. Debates about the validity of general assessments of technical efficiency (cost effectiveness) and how end-users of such guidance should interpret them need to take place.

Other technical issues that need to be addressed specifically within the framework of pharmacoeconomics include choice of outcome measurement and the design of appropriate methods for costing within evaluations. Our current means of incorporating **utility** into economic evaluations is through the estimation of changes in the quality-adjusted life-year, which is unsatisfactory for many reasons. Most new drugs bring about incremental benefits over existing therapy, even if these are only in patient convenience or acceptability. Patient preferences are becoming increasingly important and must be duly noted by decision makers.

A vital issue that is frequently not given the attention it deserves is the use of different approaches to costing healthcare. Obtaining accurate cost estimates represents essential bedrock for pharmacoeconomic analyses; without it such analyses are fundamentally flawed. Unfortunately, many analyses treat cost estimation as a simple accounting exercise. A large number of issues need to be addressed to define an appropriate costing methodology to best accord with the choices available and the **perspective** of the decision maker. The range of possible costing methods must be reviewed to identify the optimum costing methodology in the context of the study being undertaken. Much more detailed analyses of 'cost' will be required to guide cost estimates within pharmacoeconomic analyses in the future.

THE FUTURE ROLE OF HEALTH ECONOMISTS/PHARMACOECONOMISTS

It is important to distinguish the future potential role of **health economics** from the future potential contribution of the health economist. Many routine health economic evaluations will be undertaken by health professionals to compare the clinical and cost effectiveness of competing therapeutic options. The future benefits that will arise as a consequence of a growing awareness of health economics by diverse health professions vastly outweighs any potential benefits to be derived from expanding the number of health economists. The ultimate aim of health economists should be to 'do themselves out of a job' and aim to ensure that the application of health economic principles becomes second nature to health professionals and is applied routinely in their workplace. However, to achieve this, health economists will need to be visible in three areas:

- First, and perhaps most important, they must be seen as 'educators', promoting the transfer of health economics techniques to clinical colleagues.
- Second, they must be 'exemplars', showing the way to the health economic 'promised land'.
- Third, they need to be active in facilitating collaboration within multidisciplinary teams and to provide unique and valuable insights into an increasingly complex array of real-world problems.

The scientific rigour and practical applicability of pharmacoeconomic techniques and methodologies must be continually reviewed and revised if decision makers are to be more fully informed by pharmacoeconomic evaluations. Although pharmacoeconomic analyses are limited by the time constraints placed on healthcare decision making in practice, it must do so without loss of scientific credibility. If health economics were divorced from its roots in welfare economics, the discipline would lose its theoretical 'anchor' and drift aimlessly amongst a sea of applied health sciences research.

CONCLUSION

Pharmacoeconomics is a young science and needs much further development. It needs to keep its theoretical base within welfare economics and health economists need to work more closely with clinicians and other health professionals. There will be technical developments in pharmacoeconomics – some of which will be little more than fashions, some dead ends, but many will develop the science and allow it to progress. Unlike many aspects of medical science, pharmacoeconomics exists not in academic isolation but will be shaped by changes in social and economic policies. As the science improves, pharmacoeconomics will become, quite appropriately, an increasingly important factor driving health policy in the future.

REFERENCES

Great Britain Royal Commission on the National Health Service (Chairman: Sir A Merrison) 1979 Report of the Royal Commission on the National Health Service. Cmnd 7615. HMSO, London
Hughes D, Walley T 2001 Economic evaluations during early Phase II drug development. Pharmacoeconomics 19(11):1069–1077)

Appendix 1: Author's checklist for the *British Medical Journal*

STUDY DESIGN

1. The research question is stated
2. The economic importance of the research question is stated
3. The viewpoint(s) of the analysis are clearly stated and justified
4. The rationale for choosing the alternative programmes or interventions compared is stated
5. The alternatives being compared are clearly described
6. The form of economic evaluation used is stated
7. The choice of form of economic evaluation is justified in relation to the questions addressed

DATA COLLECTION

8. The source(s) of **effectiveness** estimates used are stated
9. Details of the design and results of effectiveness study are given (if based on a single study)
10. Details of the method of synthesis or meta-analysis of estimates are given (if based on an overview of a number of effectiveness studies)
11. The primary outcome measure(s) for the economic evaluation are clearly stated
12. Methods to value health states and other benefits are stated
13. Details of the subjects from whom valuations were obtained are given
14. Productivity changes (if included) are reported separately
15. The relevance of productivity changes to the study question is discussed
16. Quantities of resources are reported separately from their unit costs
17. Methods for the estimation of quantities and unit costs are described
18. Currency and price data are recorded
19. Details of currency of price adjustments for inflation or currency conversion are given
20. Details of any model used are given
21. The choice of model used and the key parameters on which it is based are justified

22. Time horizon of costs and benefits is stated
23. The discount rate(s) is stated
24. The choice of rate(s) is justified
25. An explanation is given if costs or benefits are not discounted
26. Details of statistical tests and confidence intervals are given for stochastic data
27. The approach to sensitivity analysis is given
28. The choice of variables for sensitivity analysis is justified
29. The ranges over which the variables are varied are stated
30. Relevant alternatives are compared
31. Incremental analysis is reported
32. Major outcomes are presented in a disaggregated as well as aggregated form
33. The answer to the study question is given
34. Conclusions follow from the data reported
35. Conclusions are accompanied by the appropriate caveats

Source

http://bmj.com/advice/checklists.shtml#eco

For a full explanation see:
Drummond M, Jefferson T 1996 Guidelines for authors and peer reviewers of economic submissions to the BMJ. British Medical Journal 313:275–283

Appendix 2: Checklist to evaluate pharmacoeconomic studies

1. **Is an appropriate question posed in an appropriate form?**
    A clear hypothesis should be provided, which is relevant and appropriate to the real world. It should also be possible to test the stated hypothesis within the results.

2. **From what perspective is the study undertaken?**
    Pharmacoeconomic analyses should evaluate impact of changes in resource use from overall societal perspective rather than a more limited perspective. Perspective underlying the analysis and justification of its selection must be clearly specified.

3. **Is the methodology appropriate?**
    Choice of methodology must be appropriate and is dependent on the nature of the comparison being undertaken.

4. **Is the comparator appropriate?**
    The comparator should be a reasonable alternative in the country being analysed. Reasons underlying the choice of comparator should be justified and accepted as being reasonable by clinicians.

5. **Is the evaluation based on good quality clinical evidence?**
    A critical issue underlying any health economic evaluation is the degree to which the clinical evidence is available and accurate. Ideally, the costs and benefits arising from two drugs should be compared in the same trial.

6. **Are the appropriate costs and benefits considered?**
    Perspective and methods used to measure costs and benefits must be transparent. Costs and benefits on all patients should be considered.
    Is adjustment of costs and benefits made for differential timing?
    Health economic studies should consider future costs and benefits where appropriate.

7. **Is a marginal analysis undertaken?**
    Pharmacoeconomic studies must identify the additional costs and benefits that arise as a consequence of a new (or alternative) treatment.

8. **Is a sensitivity analysis undertaken?**
   It is vital that key parameters underlying health economic analyses are subject to a sensitivity analysis.

9. **Is the analysis appropriate to the local environment?**
   It is important that local costs and methods of clinical management can be encompassed within the overall structure.

Source

Haycox A and Walley T 1997 Pharmacoeconomics:evaluating the evaluators. British Journal of Clinical Pharmacology 43: 451–456

Appendix 3: A 'crook's' guide to designing a pharmacoeconomic analysis that ensures success

This 'crook's' guide takes a light-hearted look at biases in pharmacoeconomic analyses as explained in Chapter 10 (p. 156).

1. DEFINITION OF STUDY AIM

Identify what 'outcome' our drug achieves (irrespective of how irrelevant this is to the patient's real needs) and equate this with the study aim.

2. SAMPLE SELECTION

- Inclusion criteria: preferably people who are not ill.
- Exclusion criteria: all patients that are likely to be difficult (old and ill people).
- Attitude to randomisation: – oh, if we must, but only within the small subset of patients that will benefit most from our drug.

3. ANALYSIS OF ALTERNATIVES

- Avoid head-to-head analyses unless you know that your drug will 'win'.
- Compare with placebo (for 'ethical' reasons) unless you can find a comparator that is positively harmful to patients.

4. CHOICE OF PERSPECTIVE

- Identify where the costs and benefits fall from use of our drug and exclude areas where additional costs or reduced benefits occur.
- Identify this as being the optimal perspective for the analysis of **opportunity costs** and benefits.

5. MEASUREMENT OF BENEFITS

- Equate the important dimensions of benefit to the few areas in which our drug is active.
- Choose the measurement tool (or – better still – specifically design it) to focus on our drug's strengths and ignore its weaknesses.

6. MEASUREMENT OF COSTS

- Mention the importance of using a 'marginal social opportunity cost' basis for costing (it impresses the reader) – and then ignore it!
- Blend together 'marginal' and 'average' costs from 'private' or 'social' perspectives over a 'selective' time frame to ensure that our drug looks cheaper than its competitors.
- Keep emphasising the 'value for money' provided by our drug (don't worry, nobody will know what is means, but it sounds good).

7. CHOICE OF METHODOLOGY

- If our drug is worse than our competitors, then use cost minimisation **analysis** and assume outcome equivalence.
- If it's a late-to-the-market 'me-too' drug, use cost effectiveness analysis.
- If it might exhibit some clinical benefit, use cost utility analysis.
- If it is so strange (but expensive) that we have no idea what it does – confuse them with **cost benefit analysis**.

8. ANALYSING RESULTS

- If the results do not hugely favour our drug, ignore them and redo the study with different assumptions, a different methodology and different health economists.
- Fire our in-house health economists – they obviously don't have the company's best interests at heart.

9. INTEGRATING OUR ANALYSIS INTO CLINICAL TRIALS

Don't be silly, who needs scientific validity – this is a pharmacoeconomic analysis.

10. SPECIFYING AND JUSTIFYING OUR ASSUMPTIONS

Over my dead body!

11. 'ETHICS'

- Of limited value in designing and implementing the study, but of enormous potential value in beating our customers.
- 'Now we have proven the value of our product, it is unethical (and is likely to lead to litigation) if you refuse to prescribe it despite our rational, objective and scientific arguments.'

12. CONCLUSION

- Always hint at our awareness of the limitations of the study – but then always state that such problems are due to factors beyond our control and anyway are unlikely to affect the results.
- Always emphasise in the conclusion that this pharmacoeconomic analysis has made the decision for the clinician and there is no need for him/her to further exercise their clinical judgement!

Appendix 4: Case study 1 – thrombolysis

ISSUE ADDRESSED

The Global Utilisation of Streptokinase and Tissue Plasminogen for Occluded Coronary Arteries (GUSTO) study identified a significant survival advantage of tissue plasminogen activator (TPA) over streptokinase. The economic evalua-

Issues	Assessment
i Hypothesis	The question posed is clear, well defined and important
ii Perspective	The study adequately clarifies the boundaries and focus of the study
iii Methodology	The analysis appropriately utilises a cost effectiveness framework
iv Comparator	The study addresses an important real-life choice in a head-to-head manner
v Medical evidence	The analysis is based on a large, high-quality, randomised clinical trial of thrombolytic strategies. One potential problem relates to the atypical use of tissue plasminogen activator (accelerated use over 1.5 h rather than the conventional 3 h)
vi Costs	The analysis is based upon health service charges and costs in the US. The use of such resource use and costs severely limits the applicability of such cost data to European settings
& Benefits	The quality of life analysis is incorporated. The use of telephone interviews to address the complex issues underlying the trade-off between quantity and quality of life however limits the reliability of the results
vii Timing	The analysis used statistical methods to extend 1-year survival data an additional 14 years. Such an approach requires justification because it significantly determines the level of benefits claimed
viii Marginal analysis	Incremental cost effectiveness ratios are calculated for eight clinical subgroups
ix Sensitivity analysis	Extensive sensitivity analyses were performed and 95% confidence intervals estimated
x Local applicability	Both the methods of management and costs of thrombolytic care are significantly different in the US and Europe. The results and conclusions presented are unlikely to be directly applicable to healthcare provision in Europe

tion analysed whether this survival advantage was 'worth' the substantial additional cost imposed upon the health services by TPA.

CONCLUSION

In general the focus, methodology and measurement of costs and benefits (with reservations) conformed with checklist requirements. Unfortunately, the local applicability of this study to European clinicians appears to be limited by significant variations in clinical management and costs between the health systems in the US (where the study was conducted) and Europe.

REFERENCE

Mark D B, Hlatky M A, Califf R M et al. Cost effectiveness of thrombolytic therapy with tissue plasminogen activator as compared with streptokinase for acute myocardial infarction. New England Journal of Medicine 332:1418–1424

Appendix 4

Appendix 5: Case study 2 – cholesterol-lowering drugs

ISSUE ADDRESSED

An evaluation of the cost effectiveness of using cholesterol-lowering drugs in people at varying risk of cardiovascular disease.

Issues	Assessment
i Hypothesis	The hypothesis is clearly specified
ii Perspective	The perspective of the healthcare purchaser in the UK is employed
iii Methodology	The life table approach has been widely used to assess the impact of population-based interventions. It is a valuable method of evaluating health interventions aimed at modifying the risk profile of a population
iv Comparator	The nature of the comparative analysis being undertaken is clear and well specified. A comparison with other interventions aimed at reducing heart disease (e.g. lifestyle approaches) would have been helpful
v Medical evidence	The Scandinavian Simvastatin Survival Study and the West Scotland Coronary Prevention Study represent high quality sources of evidence
vi Costs	Only a partial cost analysis is undertaken and does not consider the cost of procedures avoided, in-patient or out-patient episodes avoided or primary care consultation
& Benefits	The impact of therapy is taken directly from clinical trials without adjustment for the confounding effects that arise in real world therapeutic effectiveness
vii Timing	A 5% discount rate is used which was varied from 0–10% in the sensitivity analysis
viii Marginal analysis	An attempt is made to evaluate the marginal cost per life year saved
ix Sensitivity analysis	An appropriate sensitivity analysis is undertaken for key output variables
x Local applicability	A UK based analysis – however the representativeness of the base health authority (Cambridge & Huntington) to cardiovascular risk profiles throughout the UK is open to question

CONCLUSION

Perhaps the greatest weakness of the study is its use of efficacy data derived from clinical trials. Compliance is a major problem with long-term drug therapy and for a predominantly asymptomatic condition compliance – in practice – is likely to be significantly below the levels evidenced in trials, with a consequent reduction in the clinical benefits derived from therapy. Despite this reservation, the underlying argument that statins should be targeted at groups with the greatest baseline cardiovascular risk appears well founded and should be considered by healthcare policymakers.

REFERENCE

Pharoah P D P, Hollingsworth W 1996 Cost effectiveness of lowering cholesterol concentration with statins in patients with and without pre-existing coronary heart disease: life table method applied to health authority population. British Medical Journal 312:1443–1448

Appendix 5

Glossary

The following terms appear in **bold** on their initial mention in the main text of each chapter

Acquisition cost	The cost to actually buy the product – may be less than the listed price
Adverse selection	Market failure associated with moral hazard and often associated with health insurance
Affordability	The ability to pay for a service or item
Average cost	Total cost of a treatment or programme divided by total quantity of treatment units provided
Bootstrapping	Statistical approach used to examine uncertainty in economic evaluations
Burden of illness study	Measure of the epidemiological burden that society suffers as a result of a specific disease
Capacity to benefit	Amount of health gain likely to be received by patients
Capital costs	Costs of items that are incurred over more than 1 year, e.g. vehicles, buildings
Consumer moral hazard	Exists when patients consume more healthcare than is strictly necessary
Cost benefit analysis	CBA; economic analysis that measures costs and benefits in monetary terms
Cost containment	An approach to ensure that costs are kept low as possible, e.g. plans to reduce wasteful pre-scribing

Cost effectiveness acceptability curve	Graphical representation of the probability of healthcare intervention(s) being cost effective versus decision makers' willingness to pay per incremental unit of benefit
Cost effectiveness analysis	CEA; economic analysis that compares healthcare interventions that have a common health outcome measured in natural units, e.g. life years saved
Cost effectiveness plane	Graphical representation (in quadrants) of incremental costs versus incremental benefits
Cost minimisation analysis	CMA; economic analysis where the benefits of the healthcare intervention are proven to be equivalent
Cost of illness study	Study that quantifies the burden of a particular disease in monetary terms (direct and indirect costs can be included)
Cost utility analysis	CUA; economic analysis that usually measures benefits in quality-adjusted life-years
Decision analysis	Process that involves the explicit identification of all available choices and possible outcomes of a course of action under conditions of uncertainty
Discounting	Technique used to convert future costs and benefits into equivalent present values
Disease management	Integrated approach to treatment with the goal of improving quality of healthcare and outcomes
Drug licensing	Statutory process whereby drugs are assessed by government agencies for safety, efficacy and quality of production before they are allowed onto the market
Drug regulation	Synonomous with drug licensing
Economic modelling	A mathematical model that incorporates the costs and benefits associated with treatments to help decision makers choose cost effective options
Effectiveness	Effect of treatment when studied in real-life settings

Efficacy	Effect of treatment when studied under ideal conditions (randomised controlled trial; RCT)
Equity	Fairness; equity in health means that people's needs guide the distribution of opportunities for well-being. There are many definitions of equity (e.g. equity of access) and needs (e.g. capacity to benefit)
Evidence-based medicine	EBM; an approach to healthcare practice in which clinicians have up-to-date knowledge of the evidence supporting their clinical practice, and are aware of the strength of that evidence
Friction approach	Modified version of the human capital approach. Length of time used in the calculation depends on the time taken to fill the position again
'Gold standard'	Treatment that is widely acknowledged to be the best available or the most commonly used
Gross domestic product	GDP; total value of a country's annual output of goods and services
Health economics	Application of economics to health
Health maintenance organisation	HMO; private organisation providing healthcare to patients for a fee. Popular in the US
Human capital approach	Method for calculating the present value of future earnings
Incidence	Number of new cases of disease in a population within a specified time period
Incremental cost	Difference between the cost of a healthcare programme and the next best alternative healthcare programme
Indirect cost	Costs associated with reduced productivity due to illness, disability or death, e.g. wages
Intangible cost	Psychic cost associated with illness or treatment, e.g. pain or anxiety
Marginal cost	Extra cost of one extra unit of service provided

Markov model	Often used to model progressive illnesses, Markov models can be used to represent health states and the probability of transition among such states
Medical technology	Any medical device, drug or procedure: new technologies need careful assessment before being allowed into common use
Monte Carlo simulation	Process involving repeated simulation, each time drawing a different set of values from the sampling distribution of the model parameters, the results of which is a set of possible outcomes
Monopolist	One firm producing the goods for an entire market, holds market power
Monopsonist	Sole purchaser of goods and services in the marketplace
Opportunity cost	Cost of using resources for some purpose, measured as the benefit forgone in the next best alternative
Overheads	Often called 'joint costs' because they are difficult to link with single treatments, e.g. electricity, water, laundry
Perspective	Viewpoint of the analysis, i.e. who pays the costs
Pharmacoeconomics	Application of health economics to pharmaceuticals
Prescribing adviser	An adviser – usually a pharmacist – employed by the health authority to advise prescribers and the health authority on best quality and most cost effective prescribing
Prevalence	Total number of people with a particuar disease in a population at a specified time or time period
Producer moral hazard	See *supplier-induced demand*
Programme budgeting and marginal analysis	Technique used to allocate resources based on the premise that we need to know how resources are currently spent before we change them, and that to have more of one thing we must have less of another

Protocol-driven costs	Specific costs associated with the research itself, e.g. some of the costs of a randomised controlled trial will not be incurred in usual practice
Quality-adjusted life-years	QALY; a measure of health improvement that combines mortality and quality of life
Rationing	An alternative to allowing prices to determine the allocation of scarce resources; the same as priority setting
Reference pricing	Process of defining a reference drug (one representative of its class, e.g. atenolol for beta blockers) and matching reimbursed prices to the cost of this – usually inexpensive – reference product. If the company charges a higher price than the reference, the patient must pay the difference. Widely used in Netherlands and Germany – initially effective at containing drug costs, now much less so
Reimbursement	Processes by which third-party payers decide which drugs and medical technologies are suitable for funding
Revealed preference	Method that looks at the past decisions of individuals or policy makers to determine their preferences for certain actions/choices
Sensitivity analysis	Technique for exploring the robustness of economic evaluation results by varying key parameters in the analysis
Stakeholder	Anyone with an interest in the process, e.g. in prescribing stakeholders are patients, doctors, government or insurance agency and the pharmaceutical industry
Standard gamble	Technique that involves assessing the level of risk an individual is willing to incur to improve their health
Stated preference	The use of survey methods to ask individuals hypothetical questions about how much they would be willing to pay or willing to accept in compensation for not receiving healthcare

Supplier-induced demand	When healthcare professionals demand more healthcare for the patient than is strictly necessary
Third-party payer	Most healthcare is funded by government or by an insurance agency to whom the patient either pays taxes or a premium. The doctor and patient are the first two parties – the state or insurance company are 'third-party payers'
Time trade-off	Technique that involves asking individuals to trade-off time against improved health
User charges	A direct payment from a patient or user for a healthcare service. Might supplement the payment from a third-party payer but can also be used by a third-party payer to deter excessive use of the service
Utility	Well-being or preference that an individual or society might have for a particular health state
Visual analogue scale	VAS; scale consisting of a single line with extreme positive values at one end and extreme negative values at the other
Willingness to pay	Method for deriving preferences for treatment options/interventions based on determining what society is willing to pay in monetary terms by asking hypothetical questions

Index

Note: Bold page numbers indicate glossary references.

evaluation (*contd*)

  quality in *see* quality in pharmacoeconomic evaluation

  timing, 130–2

evidence-based medicine, 41, 71, 155

  definition, 41, **188**

exclusion criteria in cost of illness studies, 97

Expanded Disability Status Scale, 153

expectations with healthcare systems, 18

expenditure (spending) on healthcare

  equality of, 21

  international comparisons, 23, 24, 56–7

    on drugs in OECD countries, 40

  in programmed budgeting and marginal analysis, 80

externalities, 27

fee-for-service, 32

feedback to clinicians on prescribing, 44

Fieller's theorem method, 145, 149

financial cost, definition, 10

financial incentives/disincentives for prescribers, 43

financial risk, 25–7

flecainide in cardiac arrhythmias suppression trial, 150

Florida 'Healthy State' initiative, 75

formularies, 43–4

Framingham study, 150

friction approach, 95, **188**

funding

  of health services, 29–31

  in published pharmacoeconomic evaluations, sources, 48

  third-party payer decisions on (of drugs and medical technology) *see* reimbursement

gamma distributed mean, 146–7

General Practice Research Database, 90

general practitioners

  awareness of prescribing activity and cost, 44

  payment/remuneration, 32

Germany, financial incentives, 43

global issues *see* international/global dimensions

'gold standard', **188**

  in checklist for paper on economic evaluation, 158

  in cost of illness studies, 98

  randomised controlled trial as, 41

government

  healthcare responsibilities, 29, 37–42

  policy *see* policy

gross domestic product, **188**

  healthcare consumption by, international comparisons, 23, 56

guidelines

  implementation problems, 77

  for prescribers, 44

health

  defining and measuring, 8–9

  equal, entitlement to, 22

  poor *see* disease

health economics, 3–9, 17–35

  defined, 1, 3, **188**

  in drug development, 60–8, 69–70, 169–70

  future technical developments, 170–3

  literature *see* published economic evaluations

  modelling in *see* economic modelling

  post-launch/post-marketing, 68–70, 127

health economists/pharmacoeconomists, future role, 173–4

health insurance *see* insurance

health maintenance organisations (HMOs), 102

  definition, **188**

  disease management programmes and, 71, 72

  formularies, 44

health-related quality of life, data collection in phase III trials, 66

health services

  application of economic evaluation to, practical problems, 163–4

  cost of illness studies used by, 96

  funding, 29–31

  lack of competition and resource constraints within, 5–7

  national *see* national health services

healthcare

  costs, *see also* cost

  economics *see* health economics

  government responsibilities, 29, 37–42

  prioritisation in *see* prioritisation

  rationing *see* rationing

healthcare services *see* health services

healthcare systems, 17–34

  defined, 17

  economics *see* health economics

  equity in *see* equity

  evaluation, 22–4

  goals/aims, 17–19

  third-party payment in *see* third-party payment

healthy life expectancy, 92

HMOs *see* health maintenance organisations